PORTRAITS OF HOPE

CONQUERING BREAST CANCER

52 inspirational stories of strength

PHOTOGRAPHY BY NORA FELLER
TEXT BY MARCIA STEVENS SHERRILL

FOREWORD BY ROSIE O'DONNELL

THE WONDERLAND PRESS

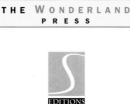

EDITIONS

DEDICATION

For Mary Jo Sherrill who underwent mastectomy surgery in Birmingham, Alabama in February
of this year with fabulous and gentle care from her doctors Viar, Ducette, and Jones, and the
nursing staff of Brookwood Hospital's Women's Medical Center, including Donna Kennedy,
Felicia Scott, Joelle Abedysian, and Winifred Dill. And in the memory of Sarah Varon Segal
who lost her battle but whose will lives on in our family.

Portraits of Hope would not have been possible without the love and support of our husbands,
François Couturier and William Kleinberg, and our children, Anabelle, Nathalie and Alexander.

S Editions is an imprint of SMITHMARK publishers.

This edition published in 1998 by SMITHMARK Publishers, a division of U.S. Media Holdings, Inc.,
115 West 18th Street, New York, NY 10011.

SMITHMARK books are available for bulk purchase for sales promotion and premium use. For details
write or call the manager of special sales, SMITHMARK Publishers,
115 West 18th Street, New York, NY 10011; 212-519-1300.

Distributed in the U.S. by Stewart, Tabori & Chang
a division of U.S. Media Holdings, Inc., 115 West 18th Street, New York, NY 10011.

Printed in Hong Kong

10 9 8 7 6 5 4 3 2 1

ISBN: 1-55670-855-6

Project Directors: Elizabeth Viscott Sullivan and John Campbell

Editor: Tricia Levi

Designer: Tanya Ross-Hughes/Hotfoot Studio

Cover illustration/design: David Hughes,
Tanya Ross-Hughes/Hotfoot Studio

S Editions thanks all of the individuals and organizations that participated in Portraits of Hope.
*This book presents the personal experiences of individuals and is not meant as a reference on the
subject. All medical decisions should be made with a physician or other qualified health professional.*

FOREWORD

Cancer. The word alone invites anxiety. When that word becomes a diagnosis, anxiety turns to terror.

Breast cancer. One woman in nine will receive that diagnosis in her lifetime. For one woman in nine the anxiety of "What if?" will turn into the terror of "What now?".

Last year, during Breast Cancer Awareness Month, I met hundreds of women, each one of whom had experienced the terror of that diagnosis. Some were in the heat of battle against the disease, their days filled with learning the language and protocols of the strange new world they had entered—awash in options, decisions, and advice, enduring the treatments and the fear, gaining strength from the hope. Some were veterans of the struggle and they survived to tell the tales, determined to use their pasts to build their futures and illuminate the present of those who must live through their same rigors. For me, it was a month of astounding inspiration. Each woman's story revealed its own particular brand of courage.

Those torrents of respect and awe overwhelmed me anew when I read *Portraits of Hope*. These women's stories reveal them as true heroes. The insurmountable surmounted. The odds defied. The sheer force of the human spirit resounds on every page. When hope is a lifeline, the generosity of those who share their stories is the ultimate act of compassion.

—Rosie O'Donnell

PORTRAITS OF HOPE

In the Fall of 1992, our Aunt Marcia was diagnosed with breast cancer, and the statistic "one in nine"—the number of women who face breast cancer in their lifetimes—was brought home to our family.

We decided that evening to embark on a mission entitled *Portraits of Hope*. Our goal was to create a book that would focus on the disease without resorting to the standard grisly images and morbid anecdotes. In pictures and words, *Portraits of Hope* tells fifty-two very personal stories in which people from diverse backgrounds reveal how breast cancer irrevocably changed their lives. While this book is resolutely positive, we never glossed over the fear expressed by each person, the pain of treatment, or the threat of death. We knew from our aunt's experience that the battle with breast cancer is terrifying, but that this disease is survivable and that the force of human will—fortified by hope—can often triumph over the disease. We wanted to present a face and voice to the inspirational battles waged every day by people with breast cancer. We also wanted this project to have a positive impact on the breast cancer cause in another important way—monetarily. That's why all of our author proceeds are being donated to NABCO, the National Alliance of Breast Cancer Organizations.

We had little idea how daunting a task *Portraits of Hope* would be to achieve. Many survivors are still reluctant to publicly discuss their breast cancer. Their reticence is a reminder of the doubly traumatizing nature of this disease—it is frightening, like all potentially fatal illnesses, but also impacts an organ tied to our perceptions of sexuality. Some survivors still feel that breast cancer treatment and surgery is viewed as mutilation and they were reluctant to open themselves up to public scrutiny. We had to coax, cajole, and reassure along the way.

Funders helped to make this project a reality: FujiFilm was supportive of Nora and underwrote film and printing costs and Myriad Gene Labs contributed seed money for the book.

Our agent, John Campbell, instantly saw the validity of *Portraits of Hope* and found Smithmark, an intrepid publishing house with a visionary publisher, Marta Hallett, and senior editor, Elizabeth Viscott Sullivan, who understood that the book's message could appeal to a broad audience. We would like to thank Rosie O'Donnell for her gracious support of this project. In addition, we would like to acknowledge the staff at *SELF* magazine and the wonderful work they do in support of the battle against breast cancer.

In an unfortunate twist of fate, Mary Jo Sherrill (Marcia's mother) was diagnosed with breast cancer as we neared completion of the project. The final manuscript was edited at Mary Jo's bedside while she recovered from a mastectomy and reconstruction in Birmingham, Alabama.

During this time, we lived through the experiences of many of the other survivors in the book. It brought home, even more profoundly, the importance of messages of hope—they do, indeed, provide inspiration and strength.

—Nora Feller & Marcia Stevens Sherrill

ABOUT THE AUTHORS

Nora Feller, an internationally published photographer, works in both Europe and America for editorial, advertising, and corporate clients, including BBDO Worldwide, Condé Nast, *People*, Forbes, Inc., HBO, *Newsweek*, ABC Television, *Town & Country*, American Express, *Elle*, Saatchi & Saatchi, *Parade*, Metropolitan Opera (New York), *The New Yorker*, and Time, Inc. She has a photography studio and home in Aspen, Colorado.

Marcia Stevens Sherrill, Nora Feller's cousin, wrote the accompanying text for the photographs, and is a frequent columnist for *Avenue*, *Country Living*, and *Peachtree* magazines. Marcia is co-owner of and designer for Kleinberg Sherrill, manufacturers of luxury leather goods and accessories. As a member of the Council of Fashion Designers of America, she has participated in the Fashion Targets Breast Cancer Project with Ralph Lauren. She appears regularly as a design authority on Lifetime Television and is currently working on a screenplay. She resides in New York City.

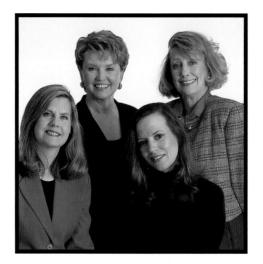

Clockwise, from bottom left:
Nora Feller, Marcia Stevens,
Mary Jo Sherrill, Marcia Stevens Sherrill

INFORMATION ABOUT BREAST CANCER
FROM THE NATIONAL ALLIANCE OF BREAST CANCER
ORGANIZATIONS (NABCO)

Breast cancer is the most common form of cancer in women in America, with close to 180,000 cases diagnosed each year. Although the means for its prevention are not yet known, finding the disease early offers the best chance for successful treatment. With early detection and prompt, state-of-the-art care, 97 percent of breast cancer patients are alive five years after diagnosis. There are two million breast cancer survivors alive in the United States today.

Each woman should have her own breast health program that includes:

• **A healthy lifestyle,** including regular exercise, following a low-fat diet and maintaining a slim weight. No smoking and use of alcohol in moderation, if at all. Research shows that these healthy behaviors may decrease breast cancer risk.

• **Regular mammograms** (breast x-rays) once a year, starting at age forty. Mammograms are safe, and can be obtained at one of more than 5,000 facilities certified and inspected by the U.S. Government.

• **A breast examination** by a doctor or nurse every year, starting at age twenty. Clinical breast exams are a complement to regular mammograms, which together find small breast cancers at their earliest stage.

• **Regular breast self-examination.** Each woman should become familiar with her breasts, and what feels normal for her. Unusual or persistent changes should be checked by a health professional.

• **Knowing you family's health history,** and discussing it with your doctor. A family history of breast or ovarian cancers, especially in a mother, sister or daughter, may mean following a different personal health plan.

The National Alliance of Breast Cancer Organizations (NABCO), based in New York City, is the leading non-profit information and education resource on breast cancer and a network of 375 member organizations. NABCO offers free information about breast cancer, including reading materials and other resources; referral to breast cancer risk, screening and treatment experts; special awareness events; and sources for financial assistance and emotional support.

National Alliance of Breast Cancer Organizations (NABCO)
9 East 37th Street, 10th Floor
New York, New York 10016
Information Services: (888) 80-NABCO
Internet: *www.nabco.org*

NABCO reminds readers that the information about each person profiled in Portraits of Hope *reflects his or her individual experience with breast cancer and resulting individual decisions about the course of care, and therefore may not reflect current medical guidelines. Decisions about breast cancer risk, detection and treatment should be made in consultation with a physician or other qualified health professional.*

Usually cast as an aggressive nonconformist, Bella Abzug radiates a calm, grand-motherly aura in her elegantly appointed Manhattan apartment. She is funny, hos-pitable, and hardly the roaring revolutionary that her detractors make her out to be. But get her talking about her latest crusade—isolating the environmental risk factors associated with breast cancer—and see the formidable warrior in her emerge.

Following a mastectomy, Abzug took her zeal for activism and her infinite energy in this new direction. She is deeply troubled by the limited funding for breast cancer research, especially for studies examining the correlation between environmental haz-ards and the increased incidence of breast cancer. "Whether you're one-breasted, two-breasted, or no-breasted, it's a two-fisted fight," declares Abzug. "Women aren't gonna stop until we find out how to prevent breast cancer and make a greater invest-ment in studying the environmental links causing it."

Bella Abzug died in March 1998 due to complications from heart surgery.

(Photographed in her New York apartment, with her hats.)

Bella Abzug

Founder of WEDO (Women's Environment and Development
Organization), Former Congresswoman

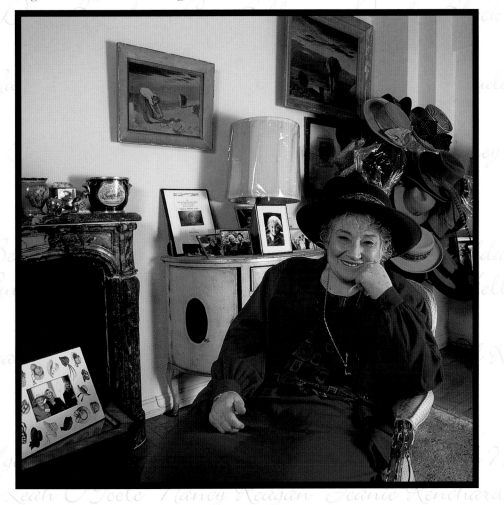

Miriam Adamson

Ms. Senior America, Professional Dog Trainer

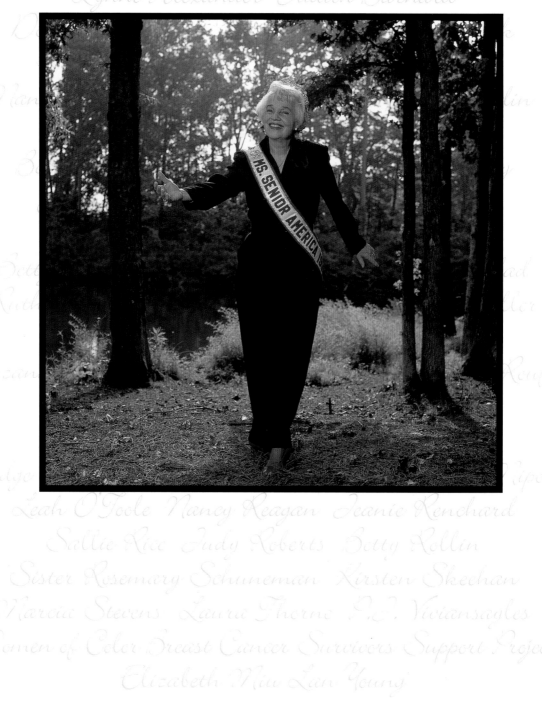

Today, almost fifteen years after her battle with breast cancer, Miriam Adamson, a former high-school literature teacher, is a walking billboard for the adage, "There is life after sixty—and then some!" She's a dog trainer, avid dogsledder, dancer, and musician.

Adamson says her life wasn't always so full. "I'm a new woman now but when my husband left me after thirty-three years of marriage, I was devastated. We raised four great kids and had a wonderful life. I truly believe that when you go through that kind of devastation, your immune system goes crazy." She feels certain that it was her state of mind that caused the cancer.

After surgery, she vowed not to be beaten, and says her high-school students saved her because of typical teenage self-absorption. They were too busy with their own lives to pander to her illness. She laughs when she recalls that though they started out with the very solicitous words, "How are you, Ms. Adamson?" the next question would invariably be, "Can I get a pass to study hall?" so they could see their boyfriends or girlfriends. When chemotherapy left her bald, Adamson picked out three wigs—one blond, one brunette, one red—and let her students vote on the color of the week. Of course, all the boys picked blond. "I was like Dolly Parton without the big breasts," she says. Adamson came through it all dancing.

Recently, a friend jokingly suggested she enter the Ms. Senior Georgia pageant. After winning the state competition, she went on to the nationals and became Ms. Senior America of 1996. When the announcer called out, "And the winner is: Ms. Georgia," Adamson was shocked. "I thought some little old lady named Georgia had won. They had to push me down the runway." What started out as a lark became more cathartic than Adamson expected. "The pageant was really a very serious matter and I loved the title and the fun of representing senior Americans. It may seem silly but I was darn proud. And all of this came after my divorce and cancer." It definitely made winning even sweeter. (Take that, ex-husband!) No longer the reigning Ms. Senior America, Adamson still enjoys the pageantry and will don the banner and tiara for a lively tap dance.

(Photographed in Marietta, GA)

Lynne Alexander gives voice to the unspoken thoughts of other breast cancer survivors when she admits she knows what it's like to be in a "morbid place," but she fought every inch of the way. She didn't even let the chemo affect her. "I refused to get sick. My oncologist couldn't believe I'd get up from the chemo and fax my lunch order over to the Carnegie Deli."

But every victory has its price. "You look in the mirror and you have no nipples, and you have a scar on top and a scar on the bottom, and you lose your toenails and eyebrows and pubic hair. Mind you, through all this, I'm trying to have a sex life!" Alexander notes, "You read about these fancy doctors and their degrees from Harvard and Yale, and you trust them, but it's about being a woman and these men think you should be thankful to them. I'm saying, 'God gave me life. Don't tell me to be happy. Happiness is not having cancer.'" Disdainful of her superstar doctors, Alexander says, "There are real issues that no one addresses. I'm tired of being sick and I'm tired of being scared, but I'm not a victim."

Alexander's mother, who lost her own battle with breast cancer recently, gave her some advice: "She told me, 'Lynne, you don't have time to worry about the cancer. You need to find a husband.'"

(Photographed at JFK Airport, New York City)

Lynne Alexander

Flight Attendant

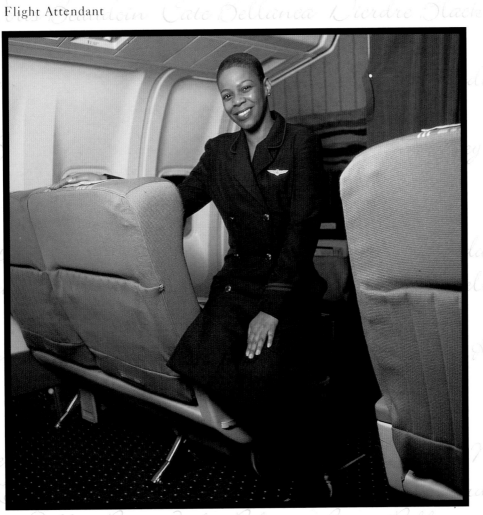

Judith Barnard

Author, with Her Husband, Michael Fain

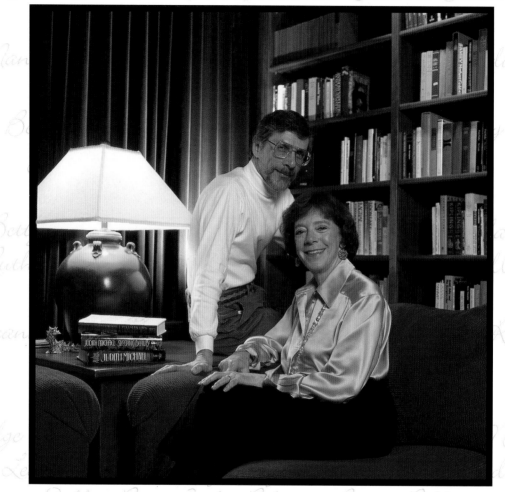

After two years as successful journalists with articles appearing in such magazines as *Redbook, Reader's Digest,* and *Ladies' Home Journal,* Judith Barnard and her husband, Michael Fain, turned to fiction. Under the shared name Judith Michael, they have written a number of contemporary novels of love, intimacy, and personal growth and self-knowledge.

"I was stunned when I discovered I had cancer," Barnard says. "I don't smoke, I breast-fed my children, I eat a low-fat diet, and I'm active in many sports." Immediately after her diagnosis, she went to Northwestern Memorial Hospital in Chicago, Illinois. Within a week she had a lumpectomy, which was followed by six weeks of radiation. "I had no effects from the radiation; it was an easy experience for me. And I never had time to be scared or even imagine dire consequences from cancer—I was too focused on conquering it."

(Photographed at their home in Aspen, CO)

Doris Beaudoin is Everywoman: wife, mother, sister, aunt, friend. Unfortunately, many women can capably juggle multiple responsibilities, but anxiety about cancer or a lack of vigilance about their health keeps them from performing the simple self-examination that can save their lives.

It was spring and the night of the banquet that signals the end of the bowling season when Beaudoin's best friend called her, scared about a lump she'd found in her breast. Beaudoin had never done a breast self-examination. She had always put it off, thinking that she'd do it the next month. Her friend's call prompted her to finally do a self-exam. She stepped into the shower that evening and came out sick. She had found a lump.

Beaudoin underwent surgery soon after. Five months later, fall found her good as new and ready for the new bowling season. Ironically, her friend with the lump did not have cancer. "Yup! She was lucky," says Beaudoin, "but so was I—I recovered and I couldn't feel better."

(Photographed at the Airport Bowling Lanes, Bloomington, MN)

Doris Beaudoin

Retired Business Owner, Avid Bowler

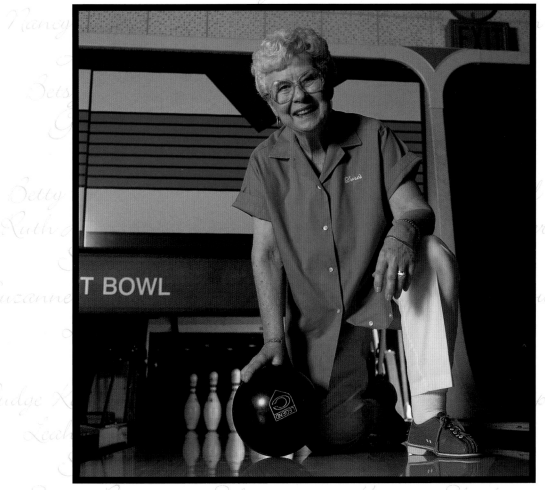

Cate Bellanca

Photo Editor

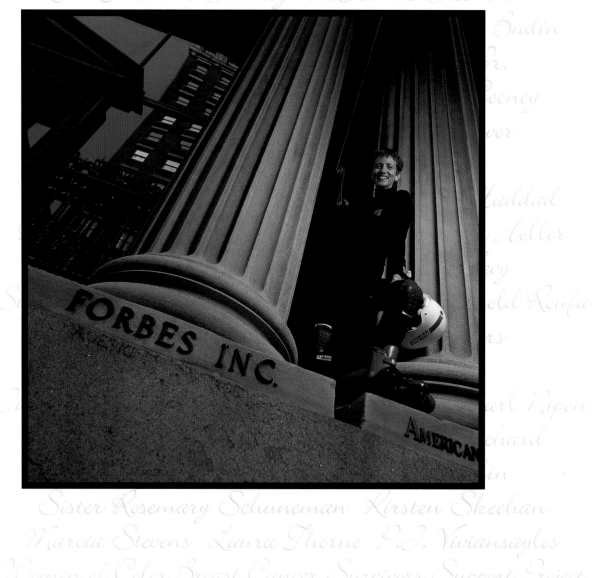

Cate Bellanca, philosopher turned photography editor, may be more comfortable discussing intellectual ideas or aesthetic viewpoints but she speaks with amazing candor about her personal experience with breast cancer.

"I was suffering from depression, and before proceeding with treatment, my psychiatrist insisted I go to my doctor for a routine gynecological exam. She wanted to make sure there were no underlying medical components to the depression," explains Bellanca. "I went for the exam and my doctor gave me such a vigorous breast exam that a discharge came out of my left breast. There was no palpable lump but because discharge can signal breast cancer, I was rushed off for a mammogram." Even though Bellanca was fortunate to have her cancer detected early, she remembers her fear and panic. "They did a magnification and showed me the cluster which was, ironically, in my right breast and not my left. They said there was a 15 to 20 percent chance of cancer. I don't know how I made it back to the office but when I got there I collapsed."

Bellanca prepared for the worst and opted for aggressive therapy—she didn't want to take any chances. "I was given a choice, but decided to have a mastectomy and reconstruction." The latter took two full years to complete. She was surprised at how complicated the entire procedure was. She elected to have a reconstruction using an implant but in order for the implant to be inserted, she had more tedious procedures to endure. "After the mastectomy heals, they insert an expander to create room for the implant and it takes several visits during which the expander is increasingly inflated with saline," Bellanca explains. She recalls, laughing, "My first expander and the scar swelled depending on the weather, so I called my breast my amazing meteorological mammary. When the implant was first in, it was also a little weather-centric but exercise and stretching have eliminated that." Bellanca credits physical fitness and a new yoga regimen with more than just quieting her internal weather forecasts. "Yoga has helped me both spiritually and physically," says Bellanca. "I'm more focused and aware of my body now and how I control my health. I felt like I needed to learn how to pay attention to my body. I've had cancer once—I don't want it again."

(Photographed at the Forbes Building, New York, NY)

A dancer since the age of five, Dierdre Black never imagined that her body, the medium and tool of her craft, would ever fail her. In 1987, the thirty-five-year-old Black was diagnosed with breast cancer after a mammogram revealed suspicious clusters that turned out to be malignant. Her surgeon was extremely cautious, though, recommending a lumpectomy without radiation or chemotherapy.

Black was in remission for two years when she had another cancer scare. Given that the cancer tends to reappear, Black was terrified and started to second-guess all of her earlier decisions. "I began to think that I should have been more aggressive the first time," she recalls. "It's all so unclear and the treatment strategies and information seem to change from year to year. When I had the lumpectomy they didn't suggest radiation and now it seems almost obligatory." Luckily, the tissue biopsy was benign.

Ten years later, Black is as physically active as ever. She's a personal trainer and massage therapist. She says emphatically of her bout with breast cancer, "It's a pretty amazing wake-up call. Life is short and I can assure you I don't waste much time."

(Photographed in her dance studio, Basalt, CO)

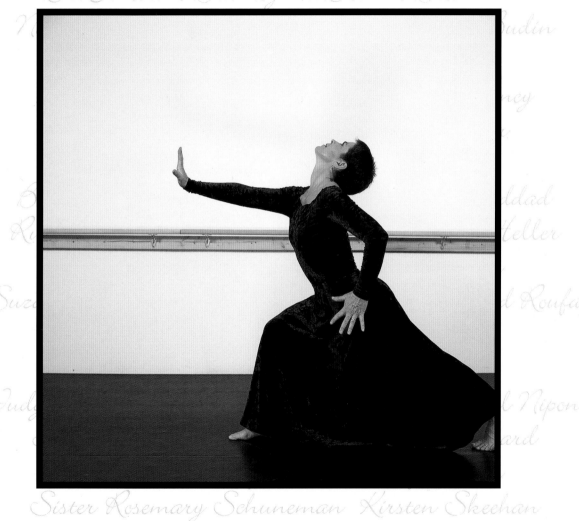

Dierdre Black

Personal Trainer, Massage Therapist, & Dancer

Bella Abzug Miriam Adamson
Lynne Alexander Judith Barnard
Doris Beaudoin Cate Bellanca
Dr. Ernestine Bradley Val Jeanne Freshman
Sudin
ncy
ldad
Heller
Suz l Roufa
Jud l Nipon
ard
Sister Rosemary Schuneman Kirsten Sheehan
Marcia Stevens Laura Thorne P.J. Viviansaigles
Women of Color Breast Cancer Survivors Support Project
Elizabeth Miu Lan Young

Dr. Ernestine Bradley

College Professor, with Her Husband, Sen. Bill Bradley

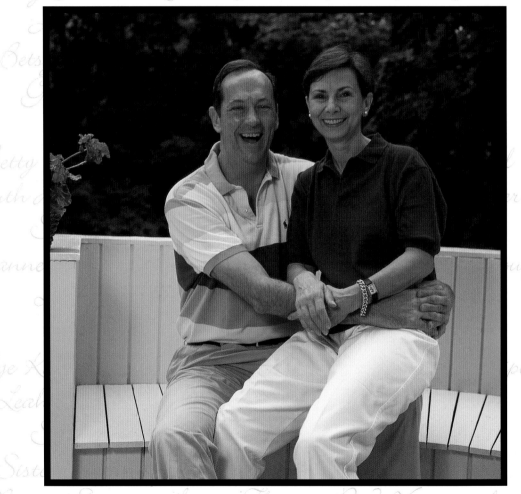

There was a time when the usually voluble Ernestine Bradley couldn't talk about her breast cancer. "It was too upsetting," she now muses. "For the first year, I didn't want to discuss it. I needed time to sort it out." Her husband, former senator Bill Bradley, took control when she was diagnosed. A compassionate and loving spouse, he became the intermediary between Ernestine and the doctors who managed her recovery. "I couldn't process all of the details and the doctors' advice. Any of it," she admits. "Thankfully, Bill was a model of support. He was there every moment talking with the doctors. He knew everything that was happening."

Of her experience, Bradley says that she "gained a sense of strength...it's difficult to grapple with the idea of mortality and for most of us it's an uncomfortable abstraction. After cancer you understand that you're mortal—it's inscribed in your body." She continues, "The inscription is postive—you are reminded that time is limited and you must make the most of it." With enlightenment comes freedom. Bradley suggests, "Cancer helps you clarify your priorities. I now allow myself more time for pleasure. I also don't agonize over trivial things, like buying new clothes. Instead of thinking, 'When will I have a great occasion to wear this?' I think, 'Life is the great occasion.'" To have battled and survived—nothing could be more life-affirming!

(Photographed at their home in Washington, DC)

ValJeanne Bresnihan can finally lift her young son, although she is recuperating from a mastectomy that is not yet the end of a long and arduous journey that began with a small lump and a tragic misdiagnosis.

In her early thirties, Bresnihan became pregnant, all the while assuming that a lump in her breast, diagnosed by her long-trusted OB-GYN as a cyst, was benign. Her doctor considered Bresnihan too young to have breast cancer. In fact, the tumor, which rapidly grew from 1 cm to over 4 1/2 cm during the course of her pregnancy (because of the surge in hormones) was malignant. After her baby was born, her coworkers urged her to get a second opinion. This time the diagnosis was cancer, and Bresnihan had an immediate lumpectomy and lymph-node dissection, and then, chemotherapy. Bresnihan thought she was in the clear but was still bitter about the experience. "I was so angry that my doctor ignored my fears and brushed them aside, even though I told him my baby wouldn't nurse from that breast and that I was experiencing pain," Bresnihan says.

Bresnihan went in for a six-month mammogram, routine for cancer survivors, and was dumbfounded by the findings—it was determined that there was more cancer and that she'd need to have a mastectomy. She had the mastectomy but is waiting to see if she'll be able to have reconstruction. An MRI showed possible bone involvement, and results from a needle biopsy of her marrow were inconclusive. Contemplating the possible grim outlook, Bresnihan says, "I have to live for my son. If it weren't for him, I wouldn't be strong enough to make it through this. He is what keeps me going."

(Photographed at their home in New York City)

ValJeanne Bresnihan

Healthcare Administrator, with Her Son, Anthony

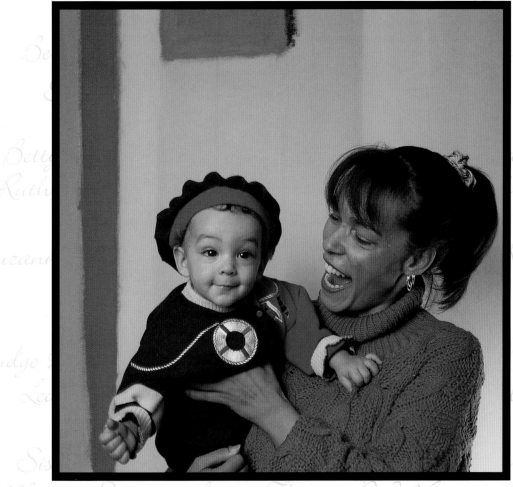

Nancy Brinker

Philanthropist, Founder of the Susan G. Komen Breast Cancer Foundation

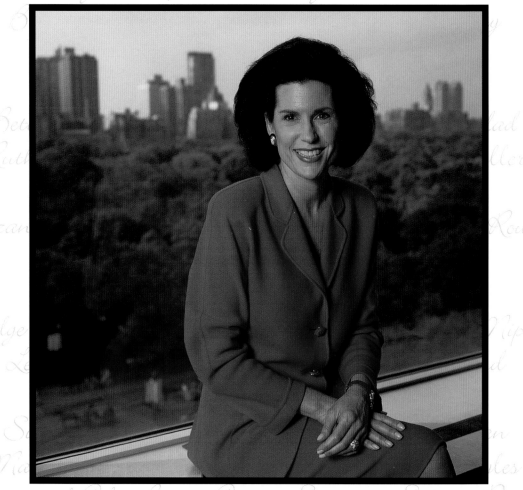

A force of nature, Nancy Brinker took her family's private battle with breast cancer and created a charity that has benefited women the world over.

Brinker and her sister, Suzy, were terrified when their aunt lost a breast to cancer. The fear it instilled in Suzy influenced many of her own decisions years later when she, too, faced cancer. Anxious to avoid aggressive treatment and a mastectomy, Suzy died three years after her diagnosis. Brinker's eventual struggle with her own breast cancer resulted in the establishment of the Susan G. Komen Breast Cancer Foundation, named after her sister. It sponsors the Race for the Cure, an annual fund-raising event that attracts hundreds of thousands to the cause.

Brinker remains a crusader and asks pointedly of women she meets: "Do you examine your breasts?" To those who claim they are too afraid to check their own breasts, she chastises, "You need to examine your breasts. What you *don't* do can kill you." Brinker is alive because she followed her own sound advice.

(Photographed in New York City)

The world record for speedy diagnosis and treatment of breast cancer may go to Ruthie Brown. She had surgery less than thirty-six hours after she first felt the lump.

Brown, a former professional cross-country skier who competed in both the 1981 and 1985 Olympic trials, faced her greatest challenge when she discovered the lump during a monthly breast self-exam. "I was in a total panic, but then I called my mid-wife." She had a mammogram immediately and scheduled an appointment with a surgeon, who performed a lumpectomy. As is the case with many women, Brown felt that a quick removal of the cancer was crucial to both her physical health and mental outlook. A week later, she decided to undergo an additional procedure—a mastectomy—for peace of mind as much as for her health. "If there was even the slightest chance that it would increase my probability of being free of cancer, then I wanted to do it," Brown explains.

Equally important for her was a simultaneous reconstruction. About reconstruction, she says, "If it can help you mentally, then it's worth it."

(Photographed in Aspen, CO)

Ruthie Brown

Philanthropist, Professional Athlete, with Her Children, Jenny and Simi

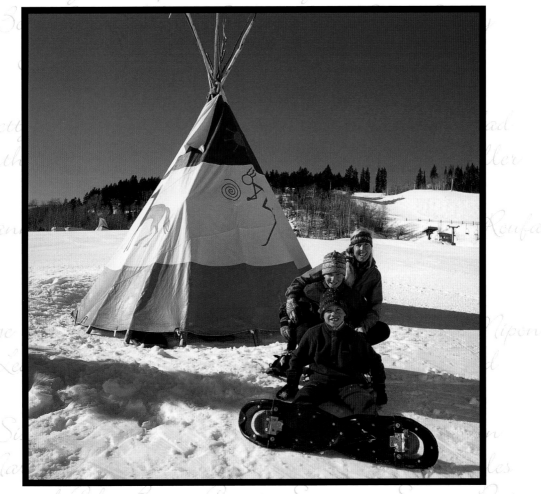

Ann Marie Budin

Farmer

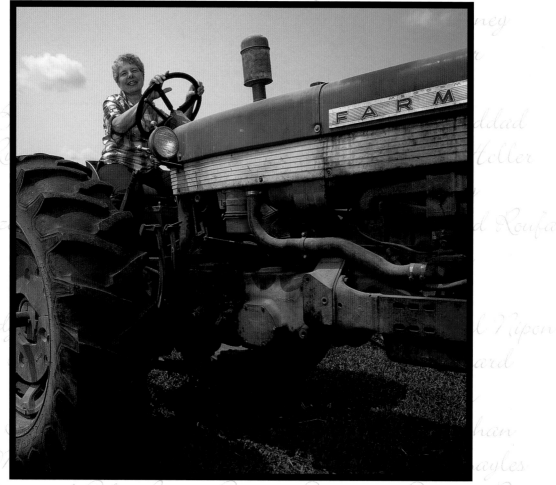

Astride her favorite tractor, Ann Marie Budin, a self-described "plain old farmer's wife," is the picture of all-American health, but in 1969, on her first wedding anniversary, she felt a lump under her arm and went to the doctor. He did a biopsy in the office but the diagnosis took several weeks because the slides had to be sent to California. Budin found out she had cancer and the surgery was performed one week after her diagnosis.

The strong-willed farmer did not take to the invalid lifestyle after the operation. She coaxed a nurse into unhooking her from the IV so she could go to the bathroom. Says Budin, "No bedpans for me. Not this gal!" When her physician heard that she had resumed her farm chores only a week after surgery, he shrugged and said, "I guess they can pick you up just as well outdoors as in, so go ahead." And on she went—and still goes on—without a moment's concession to the cancer.

(Photographed on her farm in Montgomery, MN)

Like many survivors who have been diagnosed with cancer, Judy Buie was unprepared for the dismissive attitude of many of her caregivers. However, she cherishes her relationship with Dr. Michael Moore, her oncologist, and credits him with getting her through the ordeal. "He is the most loving doctor and human being, a rare quality in what was for me a hostile experience."

Buie did not have insurance that covered routine mammography, so she went to a clinic that charged reasonable fees. The physician who broke the devastating news that the mammogram showed "something suspicious" was callous and unfeeling. He told Buie that she would need to have a biopsy. When she asked him if it could be performed there (she knew it would be cheaper), he replied, "We can do it here but there'll be a lot of blood and it's not real sanitary." She ran from the dingy office. Still shaking, Buie went back to work. Her boss suggested Dr. Moore, who had treated his girlfriend for breast cancer. "I called a lot of people for recommendations and Dr. Moore's name kept coming up," she recalls.

She went to see him. "He poked around and said, 'This is a slam dunk, a little bitty cancer, and we're just going to go in there and get it.' I felt as though I would be okay." He made the unpleasantness of going through treatment—a lumpectomy and radiation—bearable with his easy manner and optimism.

Buie advocates diligence when choosing a physician. "Find a doctor with the right personality for you. There's a very crucial mental aspect to healing, and the doctor-patient bond is going to help you heal. Trust me, I know. I'm celebrating three years of being cancer-free and Dr. Moore is a big part of my success."

(Photographed at Columbia Presbyterian Hospital, New York, NY)

Judy Buie
Photographer, and Her Oncologist, Dr. Michael Moore

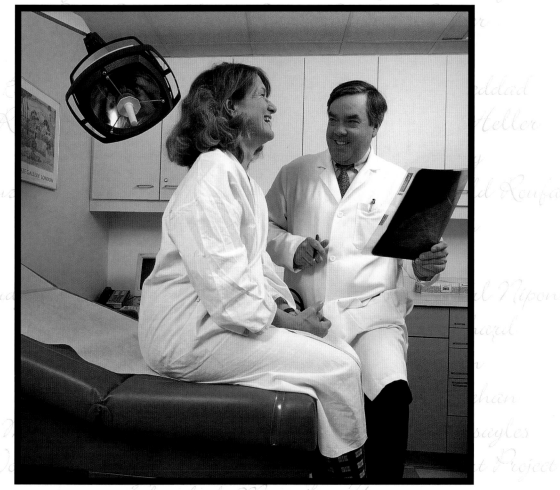

Francis "Sunny" Burnett, Jr.

Retired Postal Worker, with His Family, Latisha Rowlins,
Audrey Everett, and Gayle Burnett

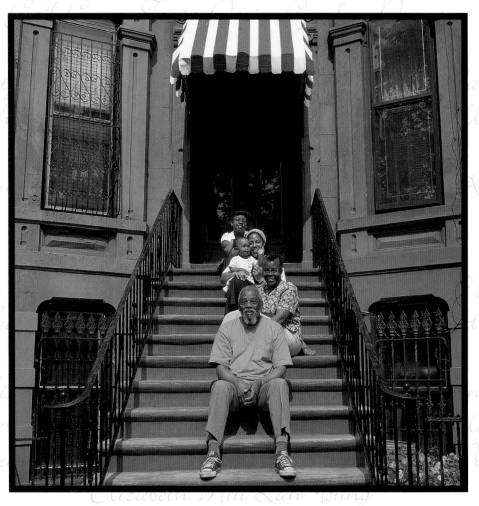

Sunny Burnett is as upbeat as his nickname implies. "I think I'm lucky," the ten-year survivor of breast cancer insists.

When he was first diagnosed, he remembers thinking, "Breast cancer? Are you sure? Wait a minute, hold on. I'm a man, not a woman." Like most men, Burnett ignored all the telltale signs, like a mysterious discharge from his nipple and pain when it was touched. Then his doctor felt a sizable lump. Although the risk of getting breast cancer is vastly lower for men than for women, it is a disease that affects both genders.

Burnett's positive attitude still holds as he battles with another round of cancer. "I've had a relapse of the breast cancer and I've been on chemo for over a year. I've had some complications from rashes so they've changed the medication three times. But I'm still up and around so don't count me out. I'll be around for a long time."

(Photographed at his home in Brooklyn, NY)

In 1992, Betsy Carter remarried, and bid farewell to *New York Woman*, the magazine she had founded in 1986, to take a chance on a freelance-writing career. Within six months she discovered she had breast cancer. Her reaction to this news was marked by her decisiveness and determination. She told her new husband and her doctor, "I want a mastectomy as soon as possible." She did not equivocate.

In addition to the mastectomy she had chemotherapy. She accepted the chemo as a life-affirming treatment and was determined not to neglect her career. During this time, Carter took on several consulting jobs for Time Warner's New Media division, started writing an autobiographical novel, and treated herself to a Hawaiian vacation to celebrate the end of chemo. "My friends joked with me that I must be taking speed, not the chemo drugs, because I got so much accomplished in record time," she recalls. "I was never so productive and I never earned as much money as I did that year—and I was freelancing."

Carter became editor-in-chief of *New Woman* in 1994 and worked there until the end of 1997. "I've always been serious about women's issues, and health has always been important in *New Woman*'s editorials," she says. "I know a lot about medicine and I am committed to keeping women's magazines on top of every advance. I'm not interested in being the breast cancer poster girl, but I definitely feel charged with a responsibility to do my bit." Taking care of herself is also a top priority. Carter plays tennis three times a week, mountain bikes, swims, and works out. "I'm physically in much better shape now than I've ever been. You could say I'm at the top of my form."

Carter is sanguine about the breast cancer. "When I wake up and it's a bleak day," she says, "I just remember that today I don't have to go for chemo. Today I don't have cancer."

(Photographed in her office in New York City)

Betsy Carter
Media Executive

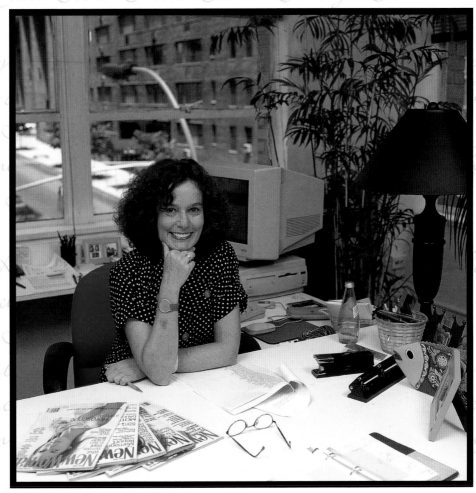

Julia Child

Author, Chef, & Television Personality

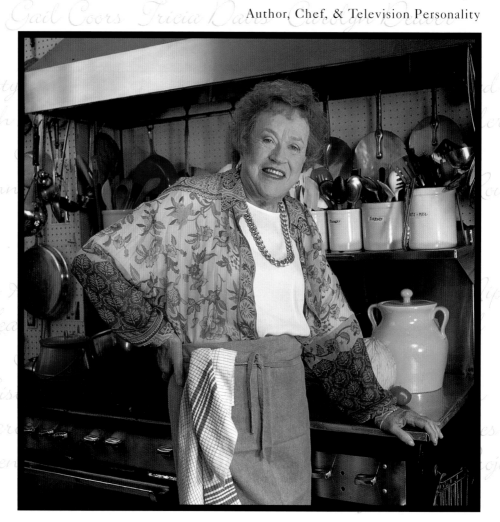

As a young woman desperately in love, Julia Child realized that the object of her desire, Paul Child, was an epicure and, as she recollects, "I was determined to get him, and if that meant cooking, so be it!" Cook she would, and if her first tentative meals were less than delicious (the marriage proposal was tendered over a humble attempt at braised calves livers), Child claims, "He did marry me in spite of my awful cooking." With her Francophile young husband, the Pasadena, California, Junior Leaguer moved to France—and it was a stint at the Cordon Bleu school that led her on a mission to popularize French cuisine in the United States. Some fifty years later, she remains the most famous chef on the planet.

Her traditionally decorated Cambridge, Massachusetts, home is filled with paintings and photographs by her late husband, the soulmate she credits with getting her through the trauma of cancer. "Paul was a dear and loving husband who anticipated my fears and reassured me. He said, 'Julia, I want you, not your breast.' Not that he didn't appreciate women's figures, mind you. But he got me through that boondoggle."

Child explains the importance of fast action. "If you hesitate to take care of your breast, once you discover a lump, you can be dead in two years. Just like that," she says, snapping her fingers. "When I found my lump, it was the size of a fordhook lima bean. I went in to my doctor and he just lopped off my breast. Whoosh! No lumpectomy, not even chemo. But my doctor always made it clear that he treats the living, not the dying."

This reminds her of how she detests the euphemisms surrounding cancer. "Oh, it's just awful. *Survivor. Victim.* I say, 'Tough titty!' Just do something about it and live."

(Photographed in her kitchen in Cambridge, MA)

Joan Ganz Cooney was a young producer from Phoenix when she cofounded the New York–based Children's Television Workshop in 1968. Seen in more than eighty-five countries, C.T.W. programs such as *Sesame Street*, have garnered some seventy Emmy Awards. Cooney herself received the Emmy Award for Lifetime Achievement and was inducted into the Television Academy Hall of Fame.

In the make-believe world of Bert, Ernie, and Big Bird, life is about facing positive challenges—counting to ten, mastering the alphabet, and learning about feelings. But Cooney didn't live in this happy world of her own making. She remembers, "I had a real double whammy. I became separated from my husband and was diagnosed with breast cancer at about the same time."

Not only was dealing with this ordeal difficult without the support of a partner, but Cooney feared that the body-changing surgery would preclude any future love life. "I remember wailing to my sister, 'I'll always be alone. No man will ever want me now.'" Her sister's reply was a classic: "Joan, you are not Marilyn Monroe. Any man who would be interested in you would never have noticed your unimpressive little breasts."

Her sister was right. Four years after her surgery, she met Blackstone Group chairman Pete Peterson at a dinner party and quickly discovered she had much in common with the former secretary of commerce.

"I could tell he was interested," Cooney recalls, "But I kept thinking, 'How do I tell him?'" She found an opportunity to broach the sensitive subject in an early phone conversation. Discussing his recent separation from his wife, Cooney cautioned Peterson to be vigilant about his health because of her view that stress can leave you open to sickness. "I said that you can get sick when you're in a weakened emotional state. When he asked me if I had gotten sick after my separation, I blurted out, 'Yes, I had cancer and a mastectomy.'" Cooney was relieved, but at the same time afraid she might have scared him off. Her worst fears allayed, they got down to the serious business of courtship, and wed in 1980.

Cooney continues to live up to her mantra: "There is no dress rehearsal in life."

(Photographed at the Children's Television Workshop studios in New York City)

Joan Ganz Cooney

Cofounder & Producer, Children's Television Workshop

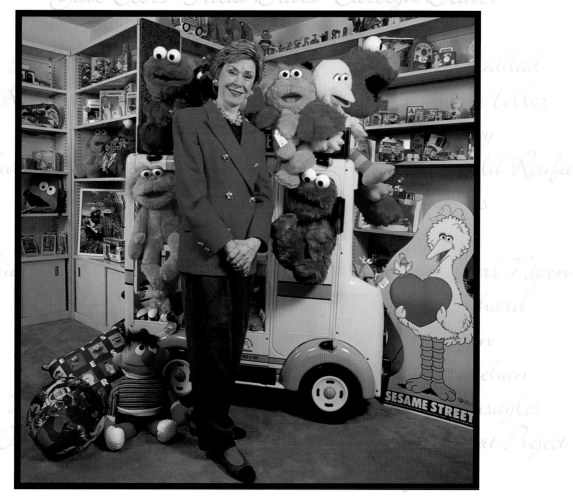

Gail Coors

Philanthropist and Activist, with Her Family

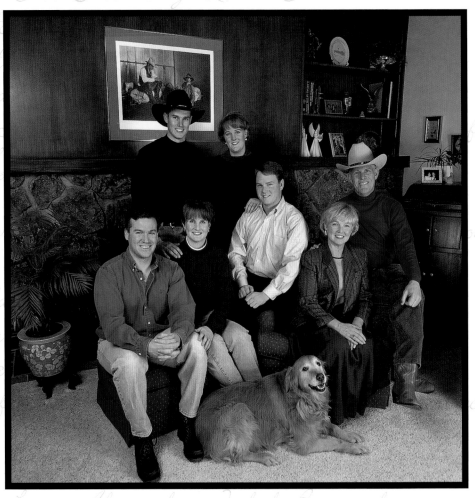

The Coorses, of brewery fame, are a tight-knit, deeply religious family. Gail Coors, the matriarch, is a dedicated volunteer in local Golden, Colorado, breast cancer charities. In the many speeches that she gives, Coors is determined to make a difference. This self-described born-again Christian has made the fight against breast cancer a personal crusade.

"My aunt had breast cancer but always said, 'My cancer has been good to me. It stayed away from my vital organs.'" Coors wisecracks, "I felt like telling her, 'You're wrong. A breast is a vital organ. If it's mine, it's vital.'" Her aunt lived until she was only two months shy of her ninetieth birthday.

Coors discovered her own breast cancer early, through self-examination. She had a mammogram and three days later a mastectomy with reconstruction, followed by an intensive course of chemotherapy. "I had every side effect you can name," she admits But her strong faith and her family pulled her through.

"My children are older and it's wonderful to have them willing to help me." Joking, Coors continues, "After all, that's the real reason for having children—to have someone to take care of you." Coors is busy these days taking care of other women with breast cancer. She volunteers and does lay counseling at her church. "I do so much work for breast cancer for the same reasons everyone else does: my mother, my mother-in-law, two daughters, five sisters-in-law, and thirteen nieces," she says. Coors knows that providing girls and women with information is vital, and that it is a gift that can mean life itself. "My girls weren't disappointed when they received how-to-do-a-self-exam shower cards in their Christmas stockings. They were thankful."

(Photographed at their home in Golden, CO)

Tricia Davis's mother, Sarah, was a model of strength in adversity. She had found her breast cancer quickly, but her lymph nodes were already involved. A radical mastectomy transformed her, leaving major indentations under her arms from the removal of her glands and breasts, and terrible scars. Unfortunately, these were very unhealthy images for her young daughter.

When her mother lost her battle with breast cancer and her own twin sister was diagnosed with it, too, Davis could no longer live with the paralyzing fear of developing breast cancer. She consulted seven doctors, investigating the possibilities of elective mastectomy. Only one of them categorically refused to perform the surgery. Other opinions ranged from, "It's valid to be considering this procedure" to "I would recommend it. You're a sitting duck."

Davis had a very real possibility of developing breast cancer because of her family history. As a result of this, she says, "The decision to have a prophylactic mastectomy was a no-brainer."

(Photographed at her home in Chevy Chase, MD)

Tricia Davis
Photographer, with Her Children, Stephanie and Ben

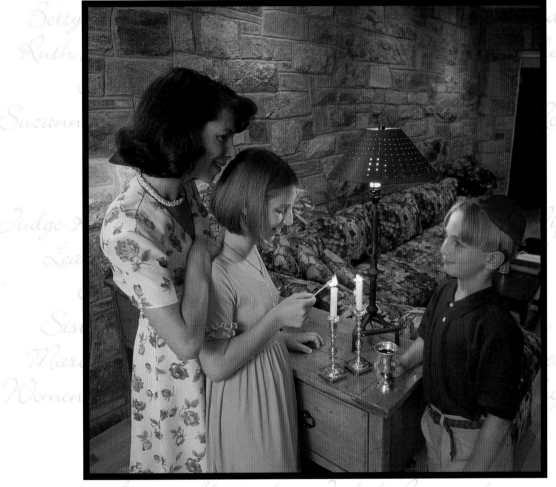

Carolyn Deaver

Vice President, Cosmetic, Toiletry, and Fragrance Association Foundation

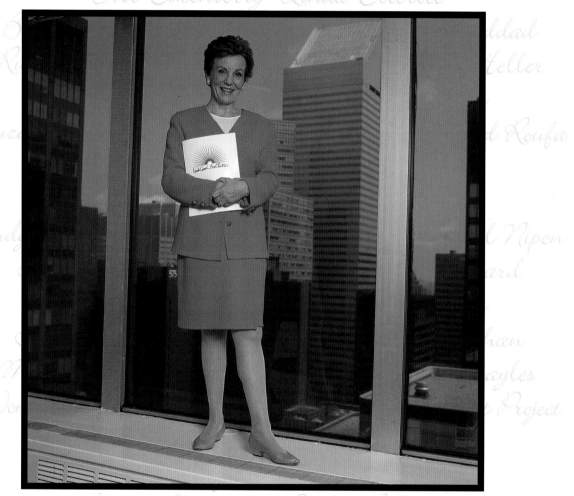

As a veteran of the Washington, D.C., political scene, including a six-year stint at the State Department, Carolyn Deaver was no easy mark for a "touchy-feely" support group. But when she was diagnosed with breast cancer in 1989, a close friend told her about the budding program *Look Good...Feel Better*® (LGFB). Though Deaver's friend didn't have cancer, she insisted that Deaver go to a meeting and get involved. Although skeptical about LGFB, Deaver finally went and found "eight women feeling the way I was—they had the same sense of loss and confusion and anger." She continues, "Other people were well-intentioned but in spite of their outpourings of sympathy I needed to know there were women out there who had experienced exactly what I had."

Deaver is now the vice president of the Cosmetics, Toiletries, and Fragrance Association Foundation which runs and funds LGFB in conjunction with the American Cancer Society and the National Cosmetology Association. LGFB sessions are held in hospitals and medical centers, the trenches of the cancer war, as well as traditional beauty treatment havens such as salons and spas.

Explaining the program's mission, Deaver, wife of ultimate Washington insider Michael Deaver, says, "*Look Good...Feel Better* teaches women cancer patients currently undergoing radiation and chemotherapy how to deal with the appearance–related physical side effects such as blotchy skin, dry skin, and hair loss, which includes eyebrows and eyelashes. Our message is that we care and understand how these women feel. We're here to offer help so that they don't lose their self-esteem and confidence." The premise is not shallow and is not a simple question of appearances. "Sometimes we are the only psychological support these women receive during the whole course of treatment. We are sympathetic, and that's a great gift. I know— I received it."

(Photographed in New York City)

In 1986, after shooting the television pilot for *L.A. Law,* Jill Eikenberry and her husband, Michael Tucker, raced back to New York from L.A. to pack up for their anticipated move to California. That's when Jill found a lump in her breast. After surgery in New York, she made time for daily radiation treatments at UCLA during the first grueling weeks of shooting the new series.

"We were incredibly lucky to get the fame and fortune, which are every actor's dream. But at the same time, we were dealing with the issues of mortality and sickness," says Eikenberry. Eventually the couple was able to turn even the negative of breast cancer into a positive dimension of their relationship. Eikenberry allows that there was a year of denial but they attended seminars and learned consciousness-raising techniques that helped them grow. "We feel as though we've gotten some marvelous tools, and we want to share them with others. That's our passion at the moment."

Traveling nationwide, the couple lecture on breast cancer and coping with it as a couple. What really interests their audiences is the "relationship stuff." Eikenberry says, "We've pulled back in terms of television, we've moved from L.A., and we now focus on working with couples who seek to love each other better through a higher level of intimacy. Our priorities shifted, and our relationship is now the priority."

(Photographed at her home in Mill Valley, CA)

Jill Eikenberry

Actress

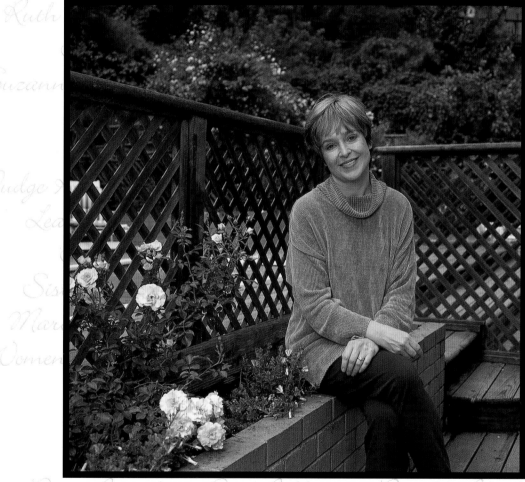

Linda Ellerbee

TV Journalist, Writer, & Producer

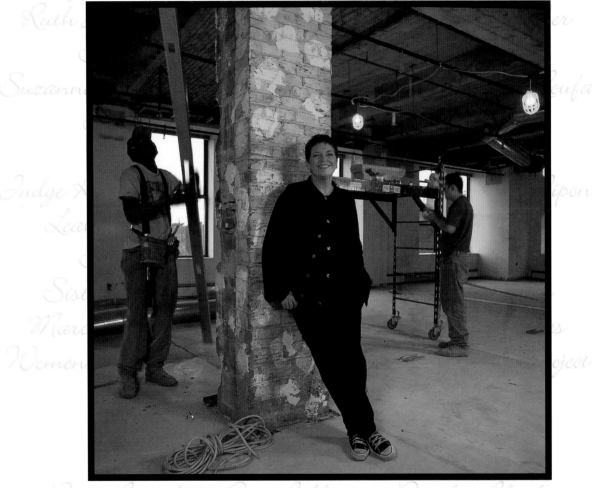

A hilarious and oft-quoted incident sheds light on how Linda Ellerbee has kept her sense of humor during her cancer experience. One day, she was playing a vigorous game of catch with her golden retriever, Bo. The frisky puppy was so caught up in the game that when Ellerbee bent over to pick up the ball and her prosthesis fell out, the dog raced off with it. A laughing Ellerbee called out to the disappearing Bo, "Hey, come back with my breast!"

Scarcely visible on the construction trolley in the background of this photo is Linda Ellerbee's talisman—a tiny stuffed duck. Purchased after an unfounded cancer scare many years ago, Lucky Duck, as he is dubbed, accompanies the energetic newswoman on all her television appearances and is a mascot for her company, Lucky Duck Productions. When Ellerbee was diagnosed with breast cancer, she underwent surgery and chemotherapy, but she has not abandoned the duck that symbolized her good fortune, nor has she lost the famous enthusiasm that has been her hallmark.

Ellerbee has earned a reputation as an outspoken, highly respected journalist whose work as a network news correspondent, anchor, writer, and producer has positioned her well to head up her own production company. She has received television's highest honors, including several Emmy and Peabody Awards, and has been recognized an unprecedented three years in a row by the Television Critics Association for her outstanding achievements in children's programming.

She is now producing children's news pieces for Nickelodeon, hard-hitting documentaries for MTV, and controversial programs on safe sex and contraception for PBS. Ellerbee brings her experience with breast cancer to bear on many of her projects. Her highest-rated documentary special for Nickelodeon, "The Body Trap," focused on kids discussing their feelings about body image and the media's role and responsibility in an image-obsessed society. Ellerbee also produced "The Other Epidemic," a prime-time ABC news special on breast cancer.

As an anchorwoman at every major network, author of two books, and mother, Ellerbee has never let cancer triumph over her spirit, and of the success of Lucky Duck, she says, "This company and our work is what I'm all about."

(Photographed during renovations at Lucky Duck studios in New York City)

While any serious illness can devastate one's family, having to endure it in the fishbowl of the White House imposes challenges beyond the personal. Former First Lady Betty Ford's revelation that she had breast cancer stunned the world. Her personal crisis made an entire nation feel vulnerable. But by the time she came through the ordeal, the world had changed, in large part because of her honesty.

Ford's decision to go public about her cancer was part of a family decision brought on by the spirit of the times in which Gerald Ford became president. "This was in the wake of Nixon's resignation, and Dad was adamant about having a completely open administration," explains her daughter, Susan Ford Bales. "We felt as if that included our family. Mother could have said she had 'female problems.' Doing what she did was tantamount to saying, 'I'm going to take off all my clothes and stand naked before you.' The hardest part for her was how people looked at her. She would meet people and they'd stare at her chest. But it really brought women with breast cancer out of the closet."

Betty Ford does not dwell on the pain. "What was most valuable to me in my own breast cancer experience was the love and support I received from my family. My husband assured me that this disease would never affect his love for me. He always made me feel whole, totally complete, and valued." Susan Bales adds, "Back then, women barely discussed breast cancer with their husbands. Luckily, Dad is different. He is cool."

With the loving support of her family, Ford paved the way for a generation of cancer patients to feel more comfortable with themselves. In tribute to the remarkable former First Lady, breast cancer advocates liken her to an avenging angel. And Bales, who carries on the family mission of combating breast cancer, is proud of her own activist role: "I have two daughters and it's a very real issue for me. I can't do enough to try to save them and all other daughters from this devastating illness."

Pensive for a moment, Ford smiles, then adds, "When I realized I hadn't thought about my cancer in over a week, I knew I had become a survivor."

(Photographed at Ford's home in Rancho Mirage, CA)

Betty Ford & Susan Ford Bales

Former First Lady and Her Daughter

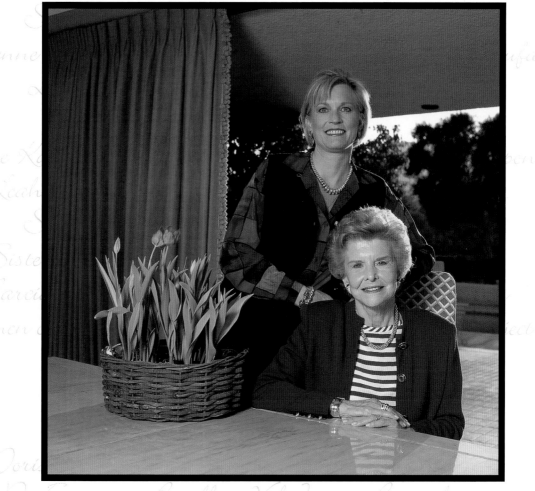

Harriet Haddad

Homemaker, and Her Daughters, Beth and Michelle

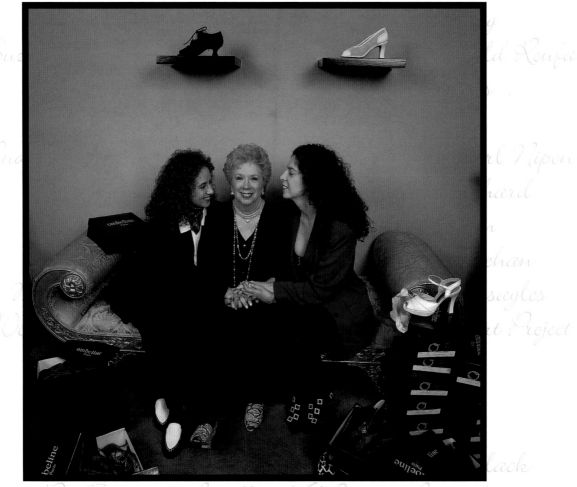

Harriet Haddad had already gone one round with breast cancer when her remaining breast was removed in 1994. Although she did not lose her hair or suffer the crippling nausea that can sometimes accompany chemotherapy, she was left with scars and an impaired self-image. She was determined to look her best during treatment and, in spite of the physical drain from the surgery and chemo, Haddad paid careful attention to her appearance. She and her daughters went to regular appointments with a beautician and shopped. She credits this positive approach with helping her persevere. "It took my mind off the cancer, got me out, and gave my spirits a boost," she explains.

A year later, Haddad opted for a double reconstruction. She is rhapsodic about the decision. "Even though it meant more surgery, I don't wake up every morning looking at these big scars. I'm not vain but it has made a tremendous difference in my life." Haddad makes it clear that reconstruction is a personal decision. "I'm not advocating it for anyone. The same goes for my feelings about estrogen replacement therapy and its role in breast cancer. I think it was a risk factor I wasn't made aware of when I started taking it. I know there are women who refute this and who prefer to continue with estrogen after cancer. I can only decide for myself. Cancer is personal."

(Photographed shopping in New York City)

In 1940, when Ruth Handler and her husband, Eliot, started their company (eventually to be known as Mattel Inc.) they never dreamed it would rack up $100 million in annual sales within twenty years—or that one of their creations, a perky, hourglass-figured doll named Barbie, would become a cultural icon the world over.

By 1966, Mattel controlled 12 percent of the $2 billion U.S. toy market, and the Denver-born Handler felt that, at age fifty, she had it all. "I had my career, my husband, my children, Barbie and Ken, and I was on top of the world."

Then Mattel began to diversify away from toys, and the company founders were caught in a downward spiral in which the Handlers would ultimately lose control. "I was diagnosed with cancer in 1970 and underwent a modified radical mastectomy. While I was recuperating from surgery, the company's problems escalated and it lost a lot of money. By 1975, after more than thirty years of building the company, I was forced into retirement."

Although her world was falling apart, Handler decided she would try to find an aesthetic and comfortable way to deal with her missing breast. "The department stores sold these fabric prostheses, these globs," she explains. "You'd feel humiliated. Here I was, a woman who had run a company with eighteen thousand employees, and I found myself timidly asking a saleswoman about the product. She handed me a surgical bra over a curtain and a wad of gloves to stuff in the bra." Commercially available prosthetics were little improvement over a cupful of gloves.

Handler discovered a prosthetist named Peyton Massey, who took a plaster cast of her good breast and made one to match. Not long afterward she had an epiphany—she would go into the breast business. She started a company, Nearly You, which developed a line of "separate lefts and separate rights" made of a polyurethane outer skin with a silicone fluid core that looked and felt natural. "My goal was to make one breast match the other side so perfectly that a woman could wear a regular bra and blouse, stick her chest out, and be proud," she says. "My other goal was to get breast cancer out of the closet."

Just as Handler was inspired to create a lifelike doll through which girls could project their dreams of being grown-up, this consummate marketeer was moved by her own experience with breast cancer to help women regain their self-esteem and sense of womanhood.

(Photographed in her penthouse apartment, Los Angeles, CA)

Ruth Handler

Cofounder of Mattel

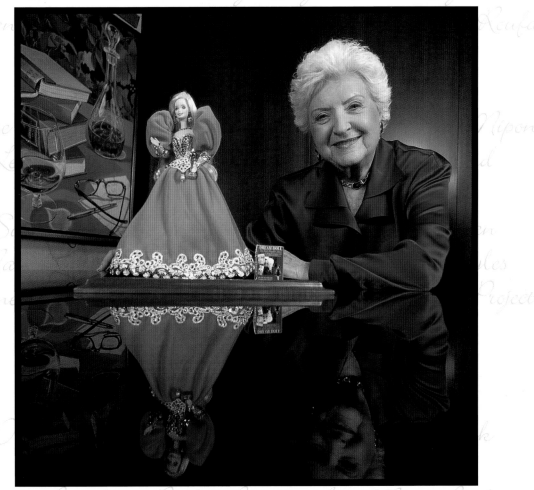

Julie Harris

Actress

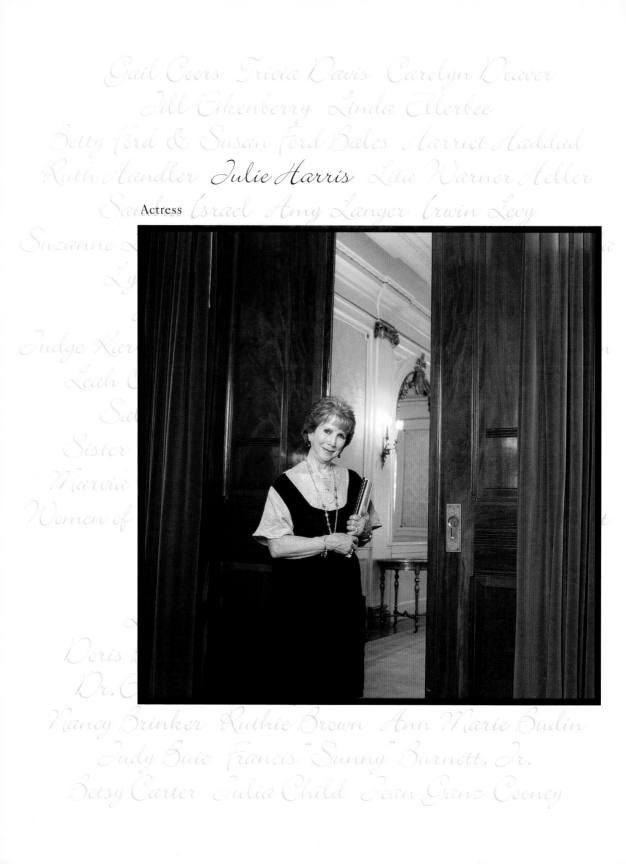

From her first movie role as the wistful child in Carson McCullers's *A Member of the Wedding* through a career that has spanned fifty years, the youthful-looking Julie Harris remains one of America's most beloved performers. Despite her loyalty to the theater, Harris was not shy about tackling Hollywood or prime-time television, and her stint on *Knots Landing* brought her international fame and a legion of younger admirers. "I had a wonderful agent, and she said, 'Just try it for a year.' I stayed seven more!" She also liked to boast that she had never missed a day of work.

Harris had been feeling fine when she discovered the lump. She was frantically busy in the early weeks of performing in the play *Mixed Couples*, with Geraldine Page and Rip Torn. Even after her suspicions of cancer were confirmed, Harris asked her physician if she could postpone the chemotherapy until after the play ended. "No," Harris recalls him saying, emphatically, her voice still sad over the loss of her role in the play, which closed soon after she left.

During her chemotherapy, Harris came across anesthesiologist Anthony J. Sattilaro's book, *Recalled by Life*, which details his own bout with cancer. Sattilaro recalls that after his diagnosis with cancer, he had been on his way home from burying his father—who also had cancer—and had picked up some hitchhikers, something he had never done before. One of them looked at Sattilaro and said, "Hey, man, you don't look so good." When Sattilaro told him that he had cancer and didn't have long to live, the hitchhiker told him about a macrobiotic diet and promised to send him a book on the subject. A few days later, the book arrived. Sattilaro read it and immediately put himself on the macrobiotic diet. Within six months, he claimed that the cancer was gone.

"Sattilaro cured himself," Harris insists. "I went on the same diet and kicked a thirty-year smoking habit. And I believed. See for yourself. I have never slowed down, and I never will."

(Photographed during rehearsal in a Beaux Arts mansion on New York City's Upper East Side)

"Life is a crapshoot, but I'm one of the fortunate ones," says Lita Warner Heller. Reluctant to play the victim, Heller has to be prodded to discuss her victorious battle with breast cancer in 1980. "I decided to have a lumpectomy. It was one of the first my doctor had performed; it was fairly early, too, in the development of chemotherapy and radiation," she explains. Heller was in the vanguard in using the then-experimental drug Tamoxifen. "I had read about it and talked it over with my doctors. I'm glad I used it—I think it did its job."

Heller has never rested on her family's laurels—her father was one of Hollywood's Warner Brothers—perhaps because she feels there isn't time. As a mother of five, a grandmother of eight, a fund-raiser for the arts, and a hostess extra-ordinaire, Heller has a long list of achievements. She was the cofounder of Les Dames D'Aspen, an Aspen charity, the former chair of the Aspen chapter of the Susan G. Komen Breast Cancer Foundation, and the honorary chair of the organization's Swing for the Cure benefit golf tournament. In 1993, she was honored as Aspen's Woman of the Year.

As for her golf ability, Heller stresses that she's hardly accomplished. "I'm just a humble beginner."

(Photographed in Aspen, CO)

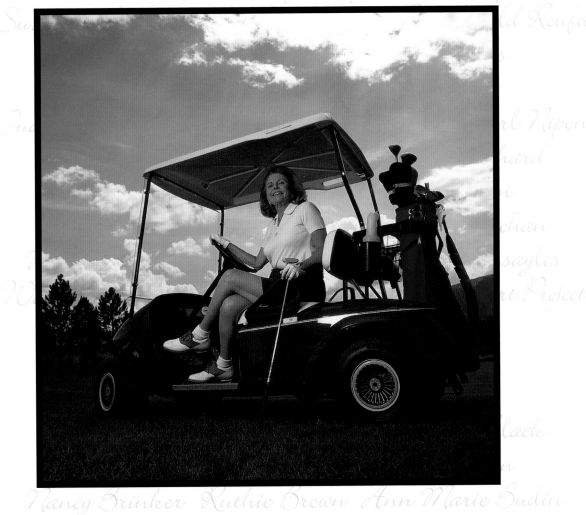

Lita Warner Heller

Philanthropist, Fund-Raiser

Sandra Israel

Fund-Raiser

Sandra Israel, an Aspen mover and shaker and eleven-year survivor of breast cancer, is very vocal about her mission, saying, "I want women to take care of themselves." As a board member of the Susan G. Komen Breast Cancer Foundation, and founder of its Aspen chapter, Israel recently initiated Ski for the Cure, a snow-capped version of the organization's successful Race for the Cure. The event attracted a glittering array of movie stars. Israel jokingly explains that "with only seventy-five hundred permanent residents living in Aspen, the celebrities have to participate or we'd have no skiers."

In addition to her year-round event planning, she also runs a support hotline for fellow cancer survivors. "What disturbs me most is the continuing controversy about the recommended age for baseline mammograms," says Israel. "When I was diagnosed at age forty-five, the insurance companies didn't cover mammograms until you were fifty. Of course, if I had waited until then, I'd be dead."

Israel remains unstintingly honest about her experience with cancer and about the arduous process of reconstructive surgery. "It's not a simple cosmetic procedure," she explains. "Reconstruction requires a full evacuation and then rebuilding."

Despite the additional surgery involved and the headline-making liabilities of silicone implants, Israel insisted on going through with reconstruction. She is pleased with her decision.

(Photographed on top of Aspen Mountain, Aspen, CO)

As a thirty-year-old senior vice president at Lehman Brothers, Amy Langer was in the midst of a large stock offering when she went for a routine gynecological exam. She casually noted her physician's remark that, with lumpy breasts, she should consider having a mammogram at some point. The appointment, which was hastily scribbled into her date book, was an afterthought, a nuisance, and Langer didn't give it a second thought. After the mammogram, she sat in the waiting room for what seemed an eternity and was then called back in for more X-rays of a suspicious lump. "It scared the hell out of me," admits Langer. "I was incredulous—thirty years old? No family history of breast cancer?" Even her surgeon was stymied—so much so that he advocated a wait-and-see approach.

Three months later, Langer decided she wanted the lump removed and switched to a new surgeon. It was a good idea—the lump was a cancerous tumor. Since this was more than a decade ago, she had to "shop around" for a lumpectomy because she didn't want a mastectomy. "I took a risk. It wasn't until a year after my lumpectomy that the definitive study came out showing equivalent survival rates to mastectomy for early-stage cancer," she explains. Not one to indulge in sentiment, Langer decided, "I was let off easily. I had my breast and I made a deal with the higher powers: I took stock of my life and left Wall Street shortly thereafter."

Although she started as a volunteer at the National Alliance of Breast Cancer Organizations (NABCO), her ingenuity helped her become the group's executive director. "I was really seduced with the possibilities of the organization and NABCO's mission. I love my job—it's intensely busy and satisfying." She also determined that all things happen for a reason: "Fate put me in a place where I can now promote positive change." Years ago, breast cancer was seen exclusively through the eyes of the physician. But times have changed. Thanks to organizations like NABCO, Langer says, "we see the disease from the patient's perspective and we are the voice of the patient." A strident voice—a voice that will be heard.

(Photographed on the steps of Congress, Washington, DC)

Amy Langer

Executive Director, NABCO

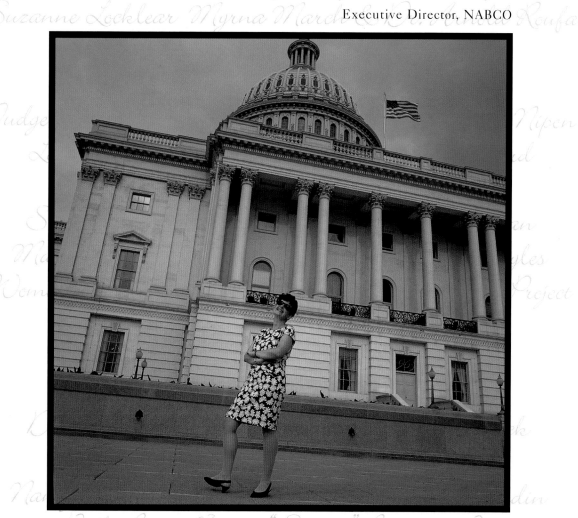

Irwin Levy
Former Professor of Special Education

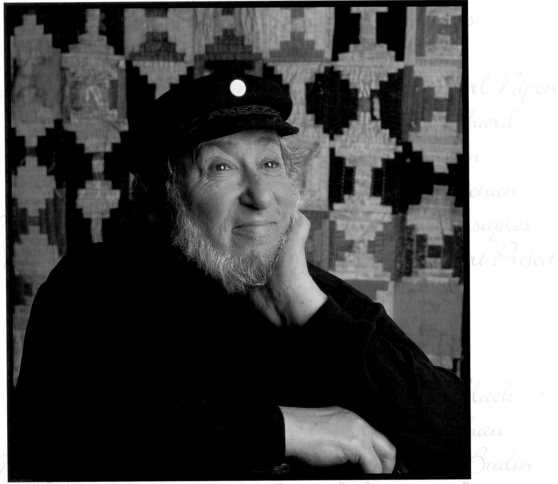

After retiring from a distinguished career in special education, the indefatigable professor Irwin Levy has undertaken an even more vigorous schedule as a volunteer, working with senior citizens and handicapped children.

Levy's nonstop energy came in handy when he was diagnosed with breast cancer in 1988. His case is a startling reminder that breast cancer does not respect gender. Sadly, it is the relative obscurity of the disease in men and the resulting lack of public awareness that often lead to dangerously late diagnoses.

Fifty-five at the time the cancer was found, Levy recalls, "If anything, it really got me angry that the cancer was interrupting my schedule and routine." His diagnosis came about by a curious turn of events. Preparing for a yard sale, he attempted to pass through a narrow doorway while carrying a heavy load, and happened to bang against the wooden frame. "I thought I had a splinter in my chest, and when I lifted up my shirt to check, I saw subtle changes in my nipple that I hadn't noticed before." The discoloration of his areola and dimpling of the surrounding skin, along with mysterious "twinges of pain," suggested that something was wrong. But like most men, he was not alert to these changes.

After two weeks, he finally went to his internist. The doctor suggested he have a mammogram. Levy was puzzled by this suggestion but the physician replied, "Don't be too shocked. Six of my male patients have had mastectomies. You haven't cornered this market!"

Levy is concerned about getting out the message that men, too, can develop the disease. An obscure PBS special with a fleeting mention of men who have breast cancer was his sole exposure to any information about the disease that nearly killed him. "All these programs are targeted at women. Men should be warned, too, and they should do self-examinations."

Cancer-free now two years after the five-year high-water mark, Levy says, "There's no way I'd let cancer slow me down. I'm just too busy for this crap."

(Photographed in New Haven, CT)

Suzanne Locklear was barely thirty when she first felt a tiny lump in her left breast. Her doctor erroneously concluded that Locklear was too young to develop breast cancer, and did not schedule a mammogram or biopsy for months, until the lump was the size of a golf ball.

When the doctor finally did a biopsy, he didn't bother to request a pathology report right away. "He just said, coldly, and probably to cover himself, 'We're going to have to remove that breast and the other one, too.' I fainted right on the table."

Her confidence in the doctor shaken, Locklear sought other opinions, which resulted in her eventually opting for a lumpectomy plus radiation, instead of mastectomy. With three small children, no medical insurance, mounting bills, and a life in chaos, she found that her marriage soon dissolved under the pressure. "I've always been an upbeat person, full of grit and determination. But things went from bad to worse," Locklear confides. She needed a job and took one selling cars. "And you know what? The man who hired me is now my husband. Sometimes when things are at their lowest point, the best moments are just around the corner. But you have to venture around that corner."

Then cancer struck a second time. Again, she followed her instincts and refused to have an immediate mastectomy. "I can be really stubborn and after all I had already been through, I felt as strong as a warrior." Locklear credits her Native American ancestry for giving her "an almost mystical understanding of my body."

"Minorities often miss out on early detection, so we have a markedly higher chance of not making it," says Locklear. Since she did make it, she has coupled her determination to create a successful business with her concerns about the lack of resources for early detection available to minority women. The result is Suzanne's Sensational Foods (Boise, ID), a line of fanciful condiments and salad dressings, she developed in 1993. She donates a portion of her earnings to various breast cancer organizations.

Locklear also counsels cancer patients locally and has cohosted a radio talk show about breast cancer with actress Jill Eikenberry (also featured in this book). "The hospitals love to send me in there to talk to patients. You know, 'Look at this woman. She's been through hell and back, but she's still here!'"

(Photographed in Boise, ID)

Suzanne Locklear

Businesswoman

Myrna March & Dr. Arnold Roufa

Former Cabaret Singer, and Her Husband, an OB-GYN Specialist

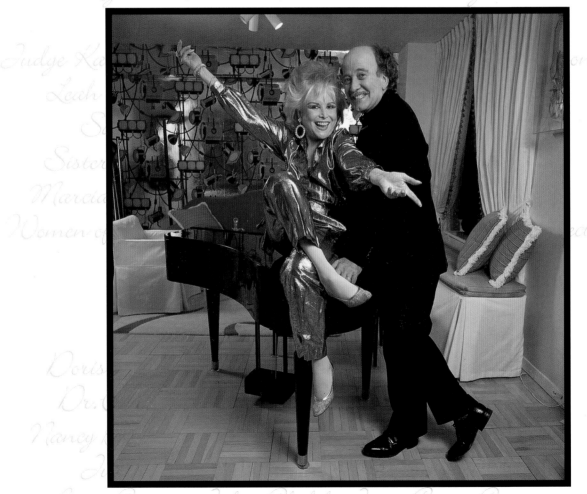

Arnold Roufa, M.D., director of OB-GYN outpatient services at St. Vincent's Hospital in Manhattan's Greenwich Village, says, "I've spent twenty-six years trying to protect my patients from cancer, twenty-two years helping my wife battle cancer, and yet I could not prevent myself from getting breast cancer." First and foremost, he is a doting husband whose every waking thought is focused on Myrna March, the love of his life.

March left home at fifteen to pursue a career in show business. She went from Hollywood ingenue to Las Vegas headliner. "I had my own TV show in Los Angeles, I was overseas with Bob Hope, I played Vegas, I sang, produced, wrote, composed—and then I got cancer," she explains.

But she says, "Cancer isn't the real killer. It's time. The doctors always wanted to wait and see, but I refused, and every time it was cancer." With a mother who died of breast cancer at the age of thirty-nine and a sister who is a survivor, March considered herself lucky to have prevailed over the disease.

March discovered the first lump in 1975 and had a mastectomy. The next year she pleaded for a prophylactic mastectomy on the remaining breast, but the practice was unthinkable. Less than a year later, she was diagnosed again with breast cancer. March laughs, "After my first mastectomy, I felt like a unicorn. The prosthesis weighed about a pound and a half and I'd have to run to put the goddamn thing on every time the doorbell rang. At least after the second mastectomy I was evened up."

While caring for his wife, Roufa developed ulcers and thought that a swelling of his breast was a reaction to the ulcer medication. He ignored it until his breast became painful even with the touch of a shirt. A short time later, he discovered that he, too, had breast cancer. A mastectomy soon followed.

In 1993 they were forced to cut short their vacation to Paris when March suddenly became ill. A CAT scan showed yet more cancer, and she continued with chemotherapy until she was hospitalized with terminal lung cancer. Now, Roufa battles alone.

Myrna March passed away in September 1997. Her beautiful smile and wonderful voice remain, along with the memories so deeply cherished by those who knew and loved her.

(Photographed in their penthouse apartment on New York City's Upper East Side)

The Al Hirschfeld caricature in this photo was commissioned to honor Lynne Meadow on the twentieth anniversary of her tenure as the artistic director of the Manhattan Theatre Club. The drawing, in which she displays that can-do, exuberant smile, recognizes her place at the apex of New York's theatre community. She's a producer and director who loves her work. "The theatre is a timeless art form that celebrates our humanity and gathers us together in a unique ritual at each performance," she explains.

Acknowledged as the most powerful woman in the American theatre when she was diagnosed with breast cancer, Meadow still never reckoned on the encouragement that she got and its importance to her recovery. She credits the "tidal wave of support from the theatre community, from the Manhattan Theatre Club, and from my fabulous women friends. They kept me alive, along with my brilliant doctor, Dr. Larry Norton. Add to that my fantastic husband, Ronald Schectman, and son, Jonathan, and my own indomitable spirit."

She was back on the stage shortly thereafter, producing *Love! Valor! Compassion!*, by Terrence McNally, directed by Joe Mantello, and starring Nathan Lane. It was a triumph and went on to become a movie starring Jason Alexander. Meadow found one of her first public appearances after being treated for breast cancer—in June 1995—a fitting climax to her experience. "I accepted a Tony Award for producing the Best Play of that season wearing a wig—and I enjoyed the celebration more than I possibly could have imagined."

(Photographed in her apartment on New York City's Upper West Side)

Lynne Meadow

Artistic Director, Manhattan Theatre Club

Millie Harmon Meyers

Press Attaché, Ambassador to the United Nations

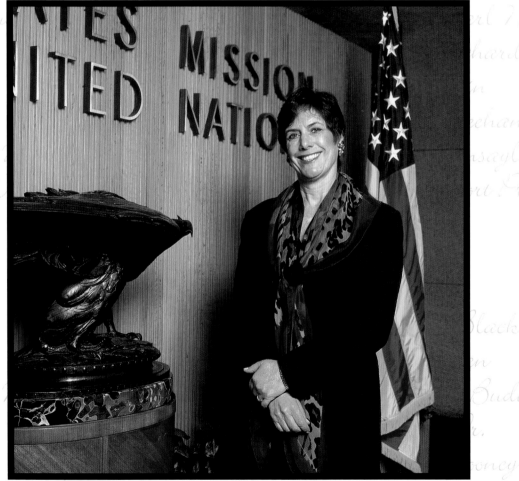

Millie Harmon Meyers was the dignified chief of protocol in the office of Madeleine Albright, before Albright became secretary of state. On a typical workday, the First Lady might have just left her office and preparations might have been under way for a visit from the president.

Her life was busy and full when Meyers learned she had breast cancer five years ago. Since her mother had battled and survived breast cancer years earlier, Meyers was vigilant about her health and had endured many nerve-racking mammograms, scheduled like clockwork. But unlike her mother, Meyers was able to choose from many options, such as mastectomy, lumpectomy, and reconstruction. She chose mastectomy, saying that the cancer was "an accident waiting to happen."

Meyers remains struck by the glaring differences between her mother's experience with breast cancer and her own. "In my mother's time, there was no follow-up. It was Russian roulette. Some survived, some didn't. And she had such horrible scarring," Meyers recalls. "My mother went to a department store to get a prosthesis and it was done so-o-o discreetly and all in whispers. Breast cancer was a very hush-hush disease back then.

She's put her experience with cancer in perspective. "I monitor the cancer, but I'm not consumed by it at all—not by a long stretch. My mother did not die from her breast cancer and that was an inspiration," explains Meyers. Facing her diagnosis with a mix of logic and intuition, Meyers says, "They didn't recommend taking the other breast but I insisted and it was lucky. When they biopsied that breast there was a small malignancy." She had reconstruction and calculates, "I've brought the odds way down for a recurrence. It's a pretty low risk, even though a cell can get away and the remaining tissue may be an issue. I take it day by day and I feel really lucky." She's also taken action. "I've made its prevention and treatment priorities. I'm on the board of the National Alliance of Breast Cancer Organizations and I'm convinced that it's critical to educate and inform women. Information is the tool that can help us make the right choices."

(Photographed at the United Nations, New York City)

Explaining the inspiration for her haunting and controversial paintings of empty bras, artist Helen Meyrowitz says, "The night before my surgery for breast cancer, I had casually thrown my bra down on the bed when the sheer weight of the image of the empty bra cup hit me."

Meyrowitz, who describes herself as a "realist with a feminist bent and a psychological undercurrent," says, "The bra took on a whole new level of meaning." From the viewpoint of composition, "the firm line of the underwire was contrasted to the soft, collapsed satin," and emotionally, "the bra's emptiness resonated." She continues, "I was scheduled for a mastectomy the next morning and I did not opt for reconstruction. I knew that when I recovered from surgery the bra would be an important metaphor." As intense as the anxiety that inspired them, the paintings have served to heal their creator—spiritually and emotionally. Meyrowitz reflects, "The panic I woke up with each morning, and the sense of loss of control and fear of death was obliterated when I got to the studio and immersed myself in my art."

No longer needing to paint the empty bras that once were a symbol of her own despair, Meyrowitz explains, "I've moved on in my art. I am now using the image of the sage fool who imparts knowledge that need not devastate." As an artist, Meyrowitz used her medium to transcend pain and panic—and to recover.

(Photographed in her studio on Long Island, NY)

Helen Meyrowitz

Artist

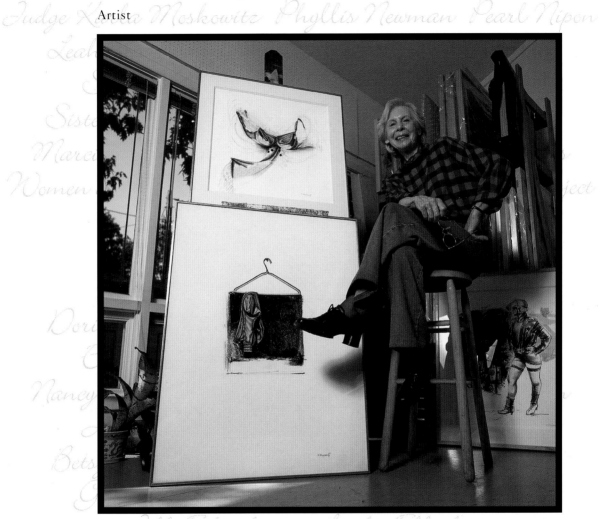

Jackie Morales

Social Worker, Activist for the Latino Community

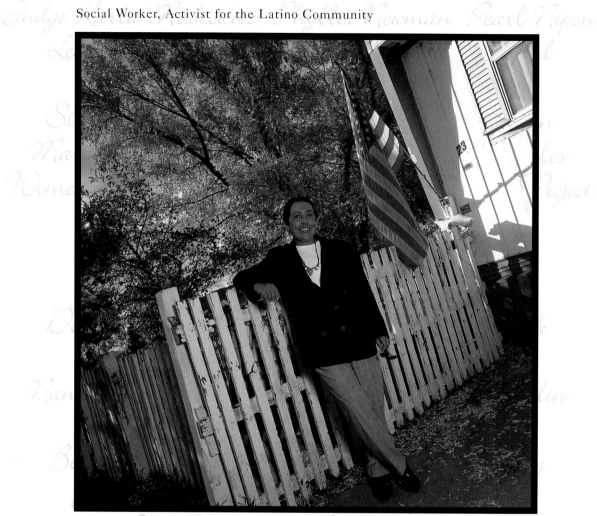

"Breast cancer is a very scary subject—but it can happen to you and it can happen to me."

These words appeared in an *Aspen Daily News* article on breast cancer, written by community leader Jackie Morales just prior to her diagnosis in 1995. "I sent the piece in, and two days later, while in the shower, I found a lump." Afterward, she felt haunted by the words she had written. Morales survived a risky bone-marrow transplant and a mastectomy in 1995. She underwent another mastectomy in May 1997.

Morales is now using her experience to help women in the Hispanic community, some of whom regard cancer as a punishment from God and a source of shame. The reluctance of certain women to confront breast cancer, and their problems accessing early-detection services, have contributed to a frightening increase in mortality among Hispanic and African-American women, as well as other minorities, diagnosed with breast cancer. Morales, a living testimonial, can assuage their fears. "They only have to look at me and it brings the message home that cancer doesn't mean death—or shame," she explains. "The community knows me and people know I'm a good girl who didn't do anything to deserve this. God is not vengeful."

Morales glows when she talks about her work despite the fact that her own prognosis is still uncertain. She has organized a local breast cancer support group and is training to be an advocate for the National Breast Cancer Coalition in Washington. In addition, she translates cancer literature into Spanish, noting that when she was diagnosed, "there was no information available in Spanish, and no one in the pictures looked like me."

(Photographed in New Castle, CO)

New York State Supreme Court Judge Karla Moskowitz recalls her bout with cancer: "I had just sent out invitations to my induction to the supreme court when my father died suddenly. After the last day of sitting shiva, I went for a mammogram. The radiologist said, 'I see something really bad. Take this film to your doctor right now.'" Judge Moskowitz remembers thinking, "This can't be happening to me. I go for mammograms regularly, because my aunt died of breast cancer. I'm vigilant—and I'd just been seen six weeks earlier by my OB-GYN."

During chemotherapy following a mastectomy, Moskowitz founded Judges and Lawyers Breast Cancer Alert (JALBCA). As copresident of JALBCA, she is involved with every aspect of the organization—from community outreach programs to mobile mammography vans, to symposiums and lectures. JALBCA is on the front line, fighting to make a difference in the battle against breast cancer. Moskowitz notes, "We've started a hotline for lawyers and judges so they can get support and information when they are diagnosed, and we educate busy professionals who, believe it or not, aren't always vigilant about self-exams and mammograms." She explains how JALBCA has helped her: "I reached out. Instead of feeling sorry for myself, I did something positive."

In her official robes, Judge Moskowitz cuts an imposing figure as she enters her courtroom. To the great fortune of those who work with her and who benefit from her dedication to JALBCA, she brings the same strength and substance that is evident in her courtroom to this important volunteer work.

(Photographed in her chambers at the supreme court in New York City)

Judge Karla Moskowitz

New York State Supreme Court Judge

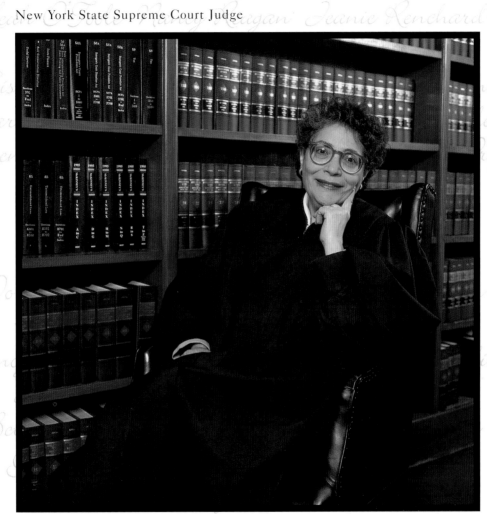

Phyllis Newman

Actress, Activist, Fund-Raiser

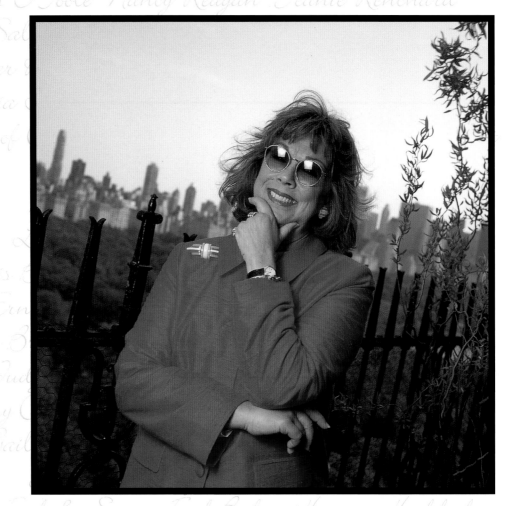

"There's No Business Like Show Business..." may well be the theme for Phyllis Newman's life. From the age of four, when she first belted out a song on the vaudeville stage, she knew her name would be in lights. She grew up on the boardwalk in Atlantic City with a fortune-telling mother and hypnotist father, and went on to star on Broadway in hits such as *The Owl and the Pussycat*, *Subway*, and *Last of the Red Hot Lovers*. She married the famous composer/screenwriter Adolph Green (*Singing in the Rain*) and has appeared on television and in movies.

Newman earned rave reviews for her book, *Just in Time*, in which she writes candidly of her battles with cancer, including two operations, chemotherapy, and her pain and fear. While never mentioning the word cancer, she recounts her panic when her health insurance expired and she had to scramble to get the requisite work (thankfully, on *The Tonight Show*) to be reinstated in the actors' insurance plan. Newman poignantly describes meeting old friends after her surgery: "The ones who hadn't seen me since the unpleasantness looked me in the eyes so straight, and so hard, that my eyes burned and hurt from their reflected intensity.... And then I counted the seconds before their eyes would dart down to my chest. Men are slower on the eye take. Women don't wait very long at all to check it out. Well, really, why should they? They're worried about their own, for Christ's sake."

And knowing that they have good reason to worry, Newman has turned back to her roots in entertainment to help other women. In the midst of a run in the hit *The Food Chain*, she launched The Phyllis Newman Women's Health Care Initiative of the Actors Fund with a benefit gala that featured Carol Burnett, Glenn Close, Kathleen Turner, and Lynn Redgrave. As Newman conceived it, the night brought together the best and the brightest. She called it "Nothing Like a Dame" and thought of it as a homecoming of sorts. "I wanted to help in the best way I knew how," she explains. "This business is my home and the people in it are my family, and we pull together in times of need."

(Photographed on the terrace of her penthouse apartment on New York City's Upper West Side)

As cofounder with her husband of Albert Nipon fashion labels, Pearl Nipon says, "I've always started my designs by thinking about how to fill a need." In 1952, when she was pregnant with her first child, Larry, she discovered that "maternity outfits were composed of two pieces: a longish top and this dreadful skirt with a big hole for your growing stomach." The Philadelphia native began designing maternity dresses of fine Italian fabrics. The dresses revolutionized fashion for expectant mothers, which in turn inspired the Nipons to branch out with a line of feminine dresses. This was a radical departure in the pants-crazed 1970s.

In less than six years, the Albert Nipon line became one of the dominant labels in the American market. Then Pearl discovered a lump in her breast. After her cancer diagnosis and mastectomy, Nipon continued her grueling schedule with weekly trips from the Philadelphia factory to the New York showroom in between chemotherapy and radiation. She was not going to let the cancer beat her. "I just kept going. Looking back, it's really a miracle that I even took the time to focus on my health. Most women don't think about themselves. I know my family and friends were probably wondering how I kept going, but the work schedule helped me get through."

For a woman who had built a career catering to the aesthetic needs of women, it was like searching for the Holy Grail to find a prosthesis that looked and felt right. "I went all the way to Germany to find something that looked natural. Remember, this was twenty-six years ago—reconstruction was very radical."

She found a good prosthesis but eventually decided to have full reconstruction. It's not the disfigurement of mastectomy that bothered her. In fact, Nipon admits, "Reconstruction doesn't work because the appearance is so perfect after having it, but because of the comfort level. You don't have to worry when you go to buy clothes. You don't have to say, 'Well, I couldn't wear this because I'd have to wear a certain kind of bra.' When I first had breast cancer, my options were: mastectomy—or mastectomy! If I'd had choices, I probably would have had a lumpectomy."

The savvy and strong-willed Nipon, an advocate for women's health choices, is a firm believer in taking control of one's life and health.

(Photographed in an Italian fabric store on West 57th Street in New York City

Pearl Nipon

Fashion Designer, Businesswoman

Leah O'Toole

Former Bodybuilder, Personal Trainer

Leah O'Toole is the picture of health. And several years ago, with her typical zest, this fitness guru met her breast cancer diagnosis head-on. A lifetime of aerobics, weight training, and belly dancing had kept her body in top form. "I was so young and vital that I felt I should do all the treatments—surgery, chemotherapy, and radiation. I knew I could withstand it," she says.

O'Toole likens chemotherapy to "drinking about ten shots of tequila back to back. I couldn't even drive. I remember trying to dial a telephone number from the doctor's office and I had to try it six times." She also went through radiation. During the treatment O'Toole felt as though her body was on "red alert" and that she had to get into a survival mode. Part of that survival mode was keeping herself fit—mentally, if not physically. She knew doing her usual workout during treatment might not be possible. "But I knew I could work out in my mind," she says. Each day she would do creative visualization. She would imagine the entire workout for an hour—each step, each lift, each crunch—and she even added new movements that helped her recover from surgery.

Taking the workout program from her head, O'Toole produced a video entitled *Gently Regain Your Range*. With an emphasis on balance and alignment, it helps the patient recover mobility and gain strength. In the video, O'Toole acknowledges the viewer's fears and limitations, but as a trainer she makes demands: "Shake it out! Put your hands on your hips. What we're doing now is arching your back and stretching your chest. Some of you may be self-conscious about sticking your chest out like this. But it's really good for you. And remember, it's just you and me in the privacy of your own home."

O'Toole is a survivor and conveys that energy to her clients. To see her smile is to feel her strength.

(Photographed at the Denver Athletic Club, Denver, CO)

Nancy Reagan has always been strong and pragmatic—as a wife, mother, and public figure—and these qualities were equally evident during her battle with breast cancer in October 1987.

After a routine mammogram revealed a small, deep tumor in her left breast, Reagan made what would become a very controversial decision. She opted for a modified radical mastectomy, although her cancer could have been treated with a less invasive procedure. She had to endure not only her private battle with cancer, but the public debate over her choice. During a *20/20* interview with Barbara Walters after the surgery, Reagan revealed that she had told her husband "I'm sorry. I'm so sorry. I'm so sorry for you," expressing the fear of many survivors that somehow they are failing their husbands by losing a breast. She also asked detractors not to criticize her for making what she thought was the right choice for her. Reagan recalls, "I couldn't possibly have led the kind of life I was leading and kept the schedule I needed to keep while having radiation or chemotherapy. If I'd been unmarried and had no children, I'd have felt differently about it." The Reagans' profound love for each other gave her the fortitude to face her frightening battle and the public scrutiny of her decision.

Today, she is sanguine about her struggle with cancer. "Whole days, even weeks, go by now and I don't even think about it. It's amazing that after something so terrifying, you can forget." She is thankful not only to have survived cancer, but to be able to enjoy life. Her family remains the wellspring of her strength, despite their very public ups and downs. "We've endured so many trials as a family that cancer seems like one of the easiest battles we ever waged. But then, that's hindsight."

Reagan's grace and dignity showed millions of American women that you can still have love and feel beautiful after cancer.

(Photographed in Los Angeles, CA)

Nancy Reagan

Former First Lady, Antidrug Activist

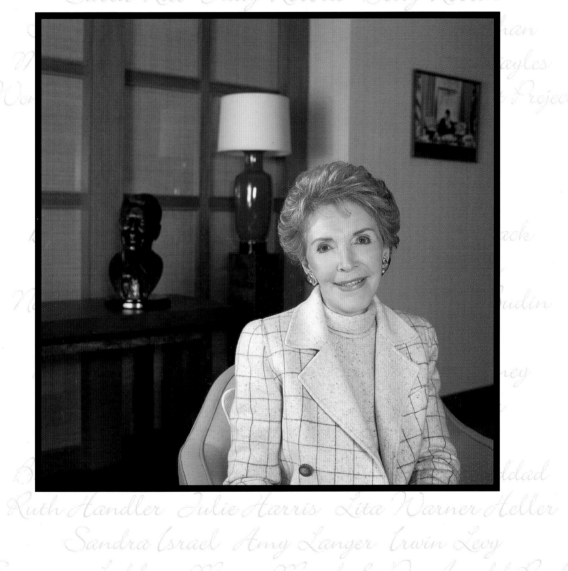

Jeanie Renchard

Artist, Horsewoman

An avid horsewoman and a celebrated sculptor of works of the American West, Jeanie Renchard was first diagnosed with breast cancer in early 1993. After serious deliberation, she chose lumpectomy and radiation. "A standard course of treatment," Renchard recalls thinking. "Perfectly safe."

But the cancer returned, and with it "a towering rage—rage at the cancer and at life." She credits her family and friends, as well as her support system of professionals, with providing the invaluable strength upon which she depended during the troubled days of her battle: "I have doctors and healers, including a psychologist, a nutritionist, a massage therapist, and a physical therapist." Together they abetted the healing process, restoring both the artist's soul and the sculptor's strength.

From Rancho Paradiso, her Rocky Mountain ranch, Renchard often writes her friends and family. "I remind them to never take life for granted and live life to the fullest. It can be snatched away at any moment. Notice every tree, every cloud, every child—and express gratitude on a daily basis." This was the mantra that guided her through the healing process.

The animals that are central to Renchard's art were paramount in her self-discovery and recovery. Her horse, Cisco, is her spiritual guide. Renchard likens him to "a pure spirit. Totally free and in the moment. I try to live as he does and make the life changes that will bring me joy." Her spiritual awakening served to strengthen her soul as she faced cancer for the second time.

To maintain her inner peace and balance, Renchard recites her own unique prayer each day:
May I be filled with loving-kindness.
May I be well.
May I be peaceful and at ease.
May I be happy.
May I be more in tune with the rhythms of nature and myself.
May I learn not to fear death.

Renchard recently completed a commission for the golfer Jack Nicklaus, entitled *The Golden Bear*—a 1,500-pound bronze sculpture of a grizzly bear. Now, with some extra time between commissions, Renchard rides her horse every day. "I am concentrating on becoming a real good cowgirl."

(Photographed with her horse, Cisco, at her ranch in Carbondale, CO)

After skipping a couple of annual mammograms, Sallie Rice, a forty-year-old corporate administrative assistant, felt a lump in her breast but did nothing about it. By the time she mustered the courage to go to a doctor, several years later, surgery was no longer an option. Her only recourse at that late stage was chemotherapy. "At the time I guess I figured I was dead, so what could they do for me? Cut it off? I'd die anyway. I stayed home waiting to die, and then I just got fed up and said, 'Well, I may keep on living, so I might as well do something.'"

Chemotherapy shrank her tumor from the size of an egg to the size of a pea, and the cancer went into remission. Rice is thankful for the life-saving chemotherapy. After her treatment sessions, she often takes a walk in Manhattan's Central Park, just as she did, dazed, following her diagnosis. "Even if you are scared and have postponed, there is still hope," Rice says, emphatically. "You just have to do something—even if you think it's too late." She feels very lucky, but cancer treatment has also come so far that even those like Rice who delay can often be saved.

(Photographed in Central Park, New York City)

Sallie Rice
Administrative Assistant

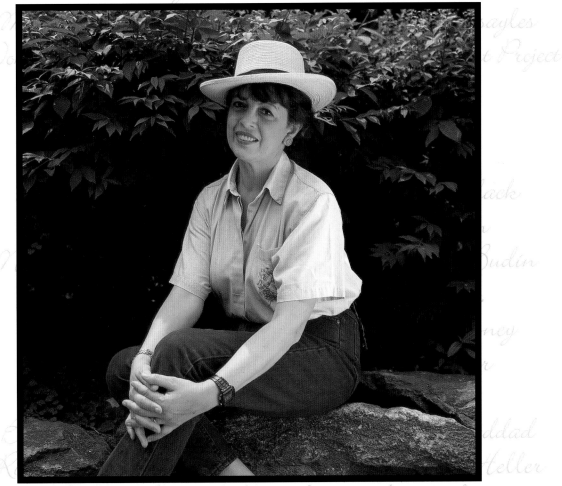

Judy Roberts

Marketing Representative

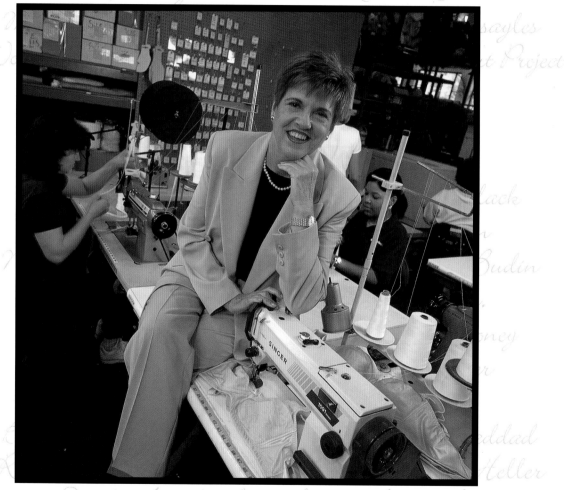

"Hey, you can be a two-breasted woman without reconstructive surgery. There are alternatives," declares forty-seven-year-old Judy Roberts with an almost evangelical fervor.

As an educator for the Amoena company's prostheses and brassieres, and user of the product, Roberts travels the world preaching to women about life after breast cancer. Roberts's message is that, although reconstructive surgery has made great strides over the years, not all women want that option. The recent debate over the health implications of silicone implants has spurred manufacturers to meet a growing demand for external prostheses that look and feel like the real thing. Today, breast prostheses have anatomically correct nipples, texture, and shape, and attach directly to the body with adhesive.

She is a classic example of a woman who refused to be railroaded into a decision. "My doctor just assumed I wanted to have reconstruction. I came to and was told I was going to have yet more surgery. I remember thinking, 'Hold on!' I knew it wasn't for me. I just said, 'Not this gal. I'll keep what I've got left and if any man doesn't want me, then God knows I don't want him.'"

"Most doctors don't even know that there is a product that can make a woman look natural, whole, and confident. They think the only way they can do that is by surgically replacing the breast. I hear women say over and over that their doctors never discussed the option of a prosthesis with them." These stories motivate Roberts in her crusade to inform not only patients but also caregivers about the options. "I've been to nurses' seminars and they'll walk past our booth with one hand over their eyes, saying, 'Thank God I don't need this.'" Roberts, exasperated, says, "Medical professionals all have their focuses. The doctor's is to get rid of the cancer. The nurse's is to get the patient through recovery. They need to see the big picture."

A born performer, Roberts loves leading her seminars. She confesses to dressing "a little sexy" and delights in fooling the so-called experts. After a lecture to a group of nurses or doctors, she routinely unbuttons the jacket of her fitted designer suit to reveal a silk teddy and no bra. She asks, "So, can you guess which one?"

(Photographed in her company's factory in Marietta, GA)

In 1974, while Betty Rollin was working as a network news correspondent, her big story was First Lady Betty Ford's disclosure about her breast cancer treatment. Within weeks of covering this story, Rollin, then thirty-eight, detected a lump in her own breast and scheduled a mammogram. The technician and doctor assured her that she was cancer-free. They were wrong, and less than a year later she had a mastectomy.

Rollin's book, *First, You Cry*, has sold several hundred thousand copies to date and was made into a television movie starring Mary Tyler Moore. In 1984, she discovered a tumor in her other breast and had another modified radical mastectomy. With her sense of humor intact, she jokes, "It's nice to have no breasts left to worry about."

(Photographed at the NBC Studios in New York City)

Betty Rollin

NBC News Correspondent

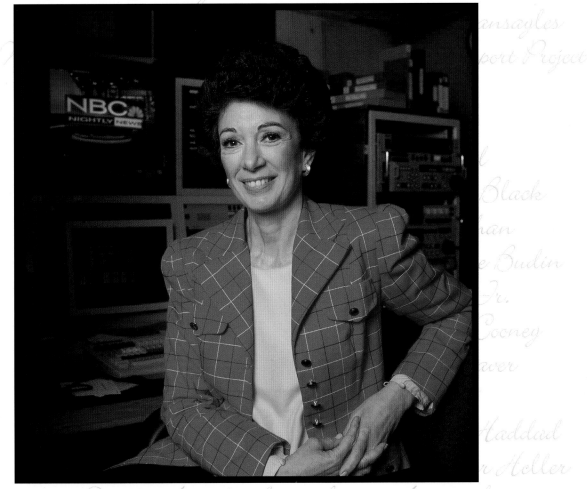

Sister Rosemary Schuneman

Catholic Nun

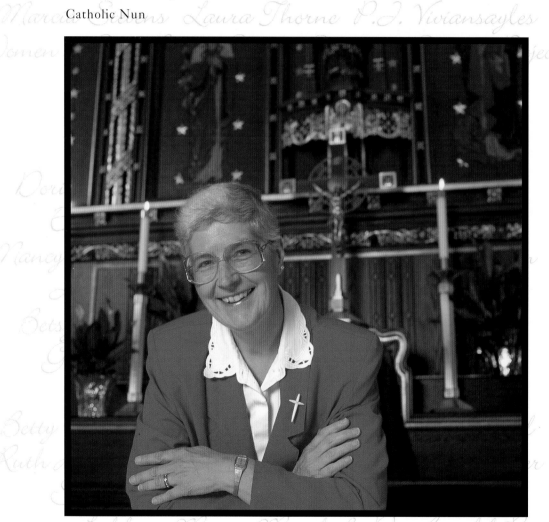

In the candlelight of St. Mark's Church in St. Paul, Minnesota, Sister Rosemary Schuneman says her rosary, grateful to have finally shed the itchy wig she wore during six months of chemotherapy. She likens the loathsome wig to the habit she and generations of nuns before her had to endure before Vatican II liberated them. "I really never felt like a woman in my habit. It takes something devastating like breast cancer, something womanly, to remind the world that its nuns are flesh-and-blood women. I like the shorter skirts. I mean, I am a woman and when I serve the community and the Church—when I serve God—I do so as a woman. I am not an 'it'."

Until about twenty years ago, nuns were seldom encouraged to be vigilant about their health. Medical concerns of a "feminine nature" were largely ignored. Sister Rosemary was diagnosed with breast cancer during an annual checkup a few years ago, and her only regret was that she agreed with her gynecologist to wait one month and watch the tumor. It grew. "I was sure they had the wrong person and the wrong test results when they told me," recalls the Minnesota native. "It was the hardest night I have ever endured. I had no family history of the disease. Nothing." She later realized that she may have been an unwitting member of a high-risk group—she has never had children and had been on estrogen-replacement therapy for more than a decade. "I am still angry that I wasn't informed about the risks of estrogen. After my hysterectomy, I was just put on it," she says.

Although Sister Rosemary is forthcoming about her experience, many in the Church still find it difficult to talk about such intimate female issues. Nonetheless, as a member of the Sisters of Notre Dame teaching order, her first step was to enlist her sister nuns in her healing. "I called on our mother house in Mankato, Minnesota, where the older sisters live. It is their ministry to pray." She believes that their continual prayer, as well as her own deeply held spiritual life, saved her. "My friends, the sisters, gave me the courage and the faith to get well, especially during the chemotherapy. It was a matter of spiritual awakening. I could feel God's presence with me," she explains. "At the end of my chemo, I had a real sense of resurrection. It was Easter, too, and after mass, my priest told me that I was glowing. I had this incredible sense of being fully alive."

Sister Rosemary constantly reminds the other nuns to take care of themselves. "I never hesitate to say, 'Do your monthly self-exam. What you don't do can kill you.'"

(Photographed in St. Paul, MN)

Kirsten Skeehan sees the irony in her battle with breast cancer. After a close friend died of ovarian cancer, Skeehan began volunteering at the Mary Helen Mauntner Project for Lesbians with Cancer, in Washington, DC. The Mauntner Project was established to address the special needs of lesbian cancer patients. "Many lesbians do not have the support structures that a straight family might provide. Many are estranged from their parents," Skeehan explains. The project works to change community perceptions of lesbians with cancer. "Doctors and caregivers need to understand that our partners want to be included. There is tremendous insensitivity out there. For example, doctors ask if a patient is married, but not if a patient has a partner. We teach women ways to avoid the trauma of coming out to their doctor."

It was while Skeehan was working as a volunteer there that she was diagnosed with breast cancer. "I needed something to do with my grief and I felt it was important to help other gay women. But after several years of emotionally draining work, I was really burnt out. I had three families who had lost a daughter or sister or partner, and it was devastating. Then bam!—I'm a client. Talk about a turning of the tables."

Skeehan's biopsy became a lumpectomy, and she went for chemo and radiation. "Chemo was okay because it's systemic. It's productive. It gets the cancer cells that have made the leap," she says. "But radiation was worse from an emotional standpoint. It's invisible, like cancer itself. They aim this thing at you and then run out of the room. Zap! Thirty seconds later, they're back. It freaked me out. But I'm here!"

She's also doing well. "My health is fabulous and life is great," Skeehan says, excitedly. "I've just returned from a year-long trip around the United States. One thing I've learned from all of this is not to postpone vacations."

(Photographed in Washington, DC)

Kirsten Skeehan

Accountant

Marcia Stevens

Communications Executive

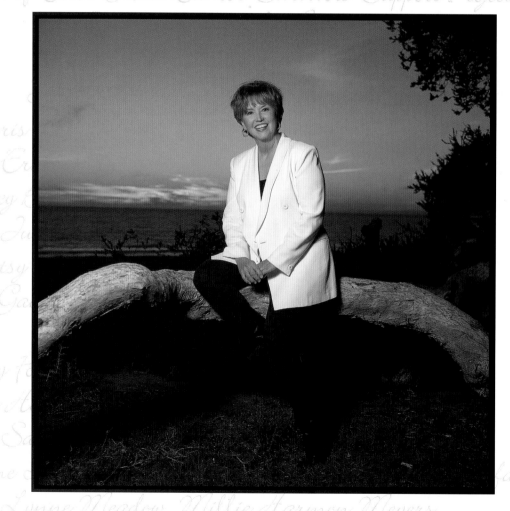

A routine mammogram picked up what appeared to be a cluster of calcium deposits in Marcia Stevens's breast. "Common enough," her doctor assured her, but insisted nonetheless that Stevens see a surgeon, just to be on the safe side. Stevens chose wisely: she hunted around and found a doctor who was a "very calm, loving, and patient James Taylor–type."

At the initial visit, Stevens was informed of her options: an immediate biopsy or a wait-and-see approach, with regular mammograms. Because her doctor felt uneasy about the cluster's configuration, they settled on a biopsy.

Three days later, the results of the biopsy confirmed her suspicions. It was cancer, but the tumor was much smaller than her doctor had suspected. He had taken enough tissue for the biopsy to qualify as a lumpectomy and was convinced that he'd gotten all the cancerous cells. "It was gone before I knew I had it."

But then the real challenge began. Stevens had been on estrogen following early-onset menopause, and standard procedure calls for discontinuing hormones once breast cancer is diagnosed. Estrogen can stimulate breast cancer's growth. "When my physician told me that I'd need to stop taking estrogen, my eyebrows hit my hairline. I wasn't prepared for feeling hot flashes again, thank you very much."

But she heeded the advice and went off hormones, trying all alternative therapies, substitute medicines, and even holistic remedies. She was miserable. "I was in a situation where I was back at work in a corporate setting, and there's nothing as frustrating as sitting in a meeting and spontaneously heating up," Stevens explains. "So, three years after my lumpectomy, with careful monitoring and a moderate risk of recurrence, I decided I wanted to go back on hormones."

Stevens was surprised by the open discussion that ensued with her doctors. "They were really great at my HMO. They assured me that I could be the one to make the decision but that I had to make an informed decision. I spent two months consulting with oncologists and endocrinologists. Although it was not their preference, they supported me in my decision and planned to monitor me more closely. They treated me like a partner in my own health care."

Her experiences have been enlightening. "I've learned a lot through all of this, not the least of which is that there are no absolutes in life and medicine is as much an art as a science."

(Photographed in Santa Monica, CA)

Six months after undergoing chemotherapy, sculptor Laura Thorne was back at work in her studio.

But she remembers the early December afternoon when she discovered her lump. "I was working in my studio and had on a heavy sweater. After working for a while I started to get hot and when I was taking off the sweater, I felt the lump. You know how you always wonder when you're doing a self-exam if you'd know? I knew instantly." She responded as quickly as possible and underwent a mastectomy and reconstruction within a couple of months of diagnosis.

Thorne, busy and enthusiastic, has sculptures in a number of important international collections. It was inconvenient enough to have to go through chemotherapy, but when her doctor warned her to stay away from her studio, that was pushing the limit: "Sculpture is a pretty grimy and messy business, and the metal dust did not complement my chemo cocktail." Rivet gun in hand, Thorne lowers her goggles and fires up the flame. "I was really lucky to have a couple of commissions with generous due dates that allowed me to return to work and get them done."

Along with her supportive family, other survivors were important in getting her through the bleak period between diagnosis and surgery. "This community of women—survivors of two years, five years, twenty years—gave me hope during my time of despair." Thinking about women who are afraid to talk about breast cancer, Thorne says, "It makes me feel sorry to realize that someone may be lonely. All of these wonderful people were there for me, sharing their experiences." The key for Thorne is to derive strength from the genuine bonds that form among women who have "been there."

(Photographed in her studio, Old Snowmass, CO)

Laura Thorne

Sculptor

P.J. Viviansayles

Founder, Women of Color Breast Cancer Survivors Support Project

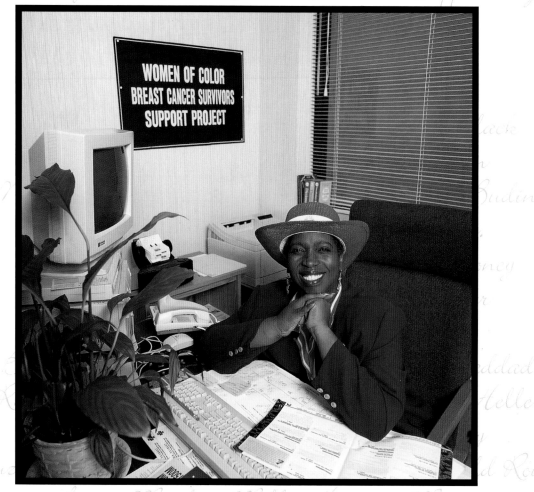

P. J. Viviansayles is the effervescent founder of the Women of Color Breast Cancer Survivors Support Project. She can spin a tale like a modern-day O. Henry and can enlist the aid of the most oversolicited corporate sponsors.

Viviansayles is a fiercely articulate champion of minority women. "African-American women's psychosocial issues are unique to their own culture and socioeconomic development. A warm and nurturing environment is needed for the survival of our African-American sisters to fight the 'silent killer' in our community."

With a grant from Avon Products, Viviansayles helped to establish the "Each One Teach One" breast health awareness outreach campaign. "Each One Teach One" has educated thousands of women at risk through its seminars. Its mantra, "Early Detection is the Key!!!" strikes a chord of hope in a community that is particularly susceptible to cancer panic.

P. J. Viviansayles died in January 1997. Through her work she charged African-American women "to participate in the advocacy of research for the prevention, early detection, and treatment of breast cancer." She was proud of her many accomplishments and kept working despite her numerous physical setbacks.

(Photographed in her office, Los Angeles, CA)

At the entrance to the Daniel Freeman Hospital in Inglewood, California, the members of the Women of Color Breast Cancer Survivors Support Project form a chain of sisterhood. Although they have not been asked to do so, they instinctively join hands for this portrait. While each woman's experience is unique, the group's very existence marks a departure from the lonely war that women of color have waged against this deadly disease.

Carolyn Tapp speaks for the entire group when she asks, "Why have all the studies been done on white women? Studies have to be done on us, too, to find answers to important questions. For example, why do we get breast cancer when we're younger? Why are we dying more quickly from the disease? Why does the disease progress faster in us?"

The women gain strength from one another. Commenting on the "Each One Teach One" program, Tapp adds, "We are trying to get the message out there. We are an underserved population." As an outreach coordinator, Tapp "visits 'womanhood' going through chemotherapy and takes flowers and fruit and remembers them and prays with them. It's comforting for them just to have women there."

Melinda Dockery remembers her relief at finding a support group for African-American women after attending a breast cancer meeting at Cedars Sinai Hospital. "All the women were elderly. Half of them couldn't walk, and I just felt like, 'Oh, no! No!' I was instantly depressed." Her experience with Women of Color has been life-affirming. "I get great rewards from it. There are women of all ages here. Every day I say 'thank you' for having found them." Dockery finds not just solace, but also some good homespun advice: When she was contending with chemotherapy-induced nausea, a friend in the group recommended drinking the pot liquor (the liquid left in the pot after cooking) from greens. "I thought, 'You've gotta be kidding! I've been suffering for four months and I could've been doing something about it?' I asked my doctor and he said, 'Well, it's not clinically proven, but I have heard of it.'" Dockery tried the potion and triumphantly returned to her doctor: "It works better than those pills you give me!"

(Left to right: Carolyn Tapp, Marylean Matthews, Gladys Jelks, Mable Laviolette Petitt Conner, Melinda Dockery, Roxie White, Grace Watson. Photographed outside the Daniel Freeman Hospital, Inglewood, CA)

Women of Color Breast Cancer Survivors Support Project

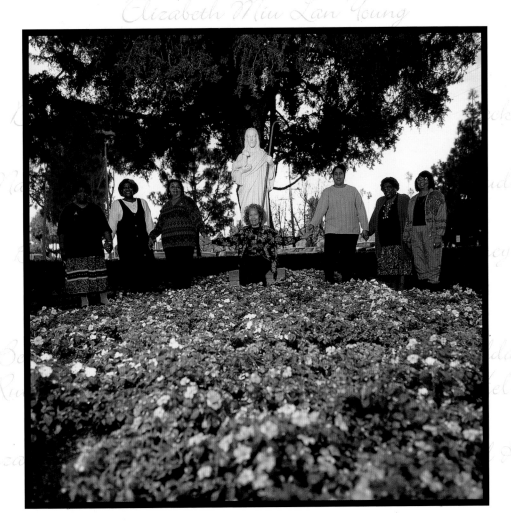

Elizabeth Miu Lan Young

Management Consultant

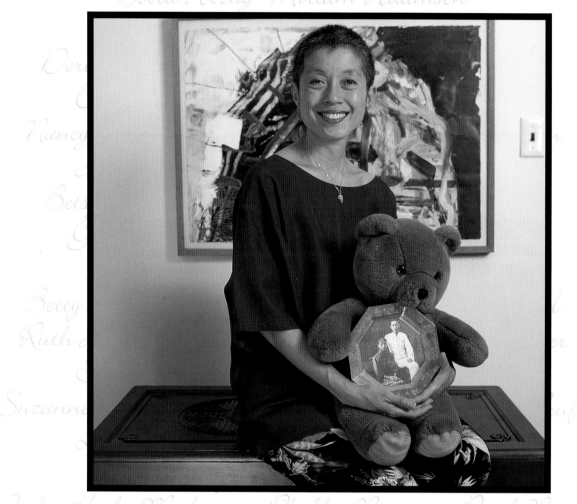

The fifth daughter of strongly traditional Chinese parents, Elizabeth Miu Lan Young has always been the family rebel. "We had conflicting expectations and values," she explains. Typical of children of immigrant parents, Young rejected their traditionalism and embraced the spirit of her 1960s youth. "You name the movement and I was involved in it," she says.

Young's strong sense of self has not only survived, but thrived, after her battle with breast cancer. "Spiritual awareness was necessary to confront my mortality. Healing is about choice, and health is the connection between mind and body and heart."

Although Young heeded her doctor's advice and underwent a mastectomy, she took control of her treatment in a number of ways. "I fought for the two-step procedure of biopsy followed later by surgery. I refused to have it happen all at once," she explains. "Many women just go under for the biopsy and then, if there's cancer, have an automatic mastectomy. I wanted to be informed about my cancer and the alternatives. The same went for the follow-up treatments."

She refused to undergo chemotherapy and radiation choosing instead to embark on a non-traditional regimen. Young's grandfather had been a Chinese herbalist, and as she explored alternative cancer therapies, she kept returning to an Eastern view of life, finding that the ways of her ancestors opened a window on hope. "I rediscovered the physical, emotional, and spiritual component to existence, where balance and harmony are the product of volition and will." Beginning with Tai Chi, which she continues today, Young pursued a four-pronged, holistic approach to healing—nutritional, spiritual, physical, and emotional—and thoroughly transformed herself in the process. "I changed my diet. I became a vegetarian and ate only uncooked foods for the first year. I also changed spiritually. I became kinder to myself. We did not have toys as children but I bought a teddy bear for myself when I had cancer. It was a comfort."

Young recently served as a facilitator at a retreat for women with breast and ovarian cancer. It was an occasion when "the teacher was inspired by the students. These women are amazingly powerful. I was struck by their strength and will to survive, and desire to help one another. Their sense of community was overwhelming and I felt at home."

For Young, breast cancer was a catalyst. "My cancer gave me the courage to say yes to life and no to unhappiness, which included leaving behind an unhappy marriage. I chose to live."

(Photographed in her apartment on New York City's Upper West Side)

ACKNOWLEDGMENTS

CORPORATE SPONSORS:
Fuji Photo Film, USA
Myriad Gene Labs, Salt Lake City, Utah
Coloplast Corporation, Amoena Prosthetics Division, Marietta, Georgia
Suzanne's Sensational Foods, Boise, Idaho
Forbes, Inc., New York, New York
Founders Funds, Denver, Colorado

PRIVATE SPONSORS:
Westside Tennis Club and Members, Forest Hills, New York
Diane Jenkins
Ethel Romano
3 Melrose Place Salon, Los Angeles, California

SPECIAL THANKS TO:
Our Photography Assistants: Angela Balduf and Elizabeth Romano
Our Agent: John Campbell
Carlos and Missy Falchi without whom this book would not be possible
Creative Vision: Carey Adina Karmel
Our Editors: Laura Fisher-Kaiser and Pamela Rendsland
Author Photographer (image, page 6): Bill Westheimer
Makeup Artist (image, page 6): Soohee Lee

OUR DEEPEST GRATITUDE TO:
Susan Ackerman, Catherine Bellanca, Janie Bennett, Mislin Bontiff,
Laurie Brant, Jerry Brennen, Sherry Bruff, Earl Crittenden, Louise Daniels-Miller,
Jessica Dewitt, Ben Diep, Alexandra Drew, Deborah & Denise Esposito,
Jerilyne & David Evenskaas, Karin Grant, Sarah Harris, Mary Hayes,
Julie Hiltunen, Joie Jones, Sylvia & Steven Kay, Bonnie Kirschstein,
Alice Kleinberg, Kevin Knaus, Carole Lalli, Dr. Barbara Landreth, Amy Langer,
Hilary Lewis, Nancy Lovendahl, Nathalie Martin-Schettini, Dr. Hannae Meiland,
Frank Micelotta, Christine Monteith, Janet O'Grady, Deborah Pierce, Crary Pullen,
Terri Rea, Karen Regan, Ethel & Elie Romano, Doris L. Sassower,
Jason Schneider, Dr. Nathan Segal, William Sherrill, Jeffrey Shotwell,
Don Springer, Sheila Tate, John Thornton, Sandy Thurman, Marianne Townsend,
Alison Wagner, Jeanette Warner, Bill and Lisa Westheimer